Table of Conter...

Preface

Introduction

Principle #**1** : Quality

Resources

Tables

PREFACE

The secret about losing weight and getting lean is that there is no **secret!** As you will see, getting lean happens when you adhere to a specific lifestyle and apply specific strategies related to food. It's all about:

Quality, Quantity and Timing!

The Story

As a physical therapist, I am fortunate to have a wealth of knowledge about movement, exercise, and injury prevention. Unfortunately diet was never something I completely understood. Although I would exercise, I was always overweight. Any time I did lose weight I felt tired and looked thin and flabby. Frankly, I was kind of embarrassed that at the age of 39, I still had no idea how to permanently and effectively manage my weight and my body composition. Worse, my wife and I were responsible to teach our children how and what to eat.

In May of 2013, I had the opportunity to treat a patient who was a professional body builder, and a successful one at that. Several years before I knew him, he was crowned Mr. New Jersey. Now, I don't necessarily condone all the behavior in that sport, but for one thing, he knew how to get lean.

On one occasion I asked him, " Why, when I lose weight, I feel tired and lose all my muscle instead of getting lean and feeling healthy? What's the secret?" His answer was simple. **"It's your diet. It's all wrong."** Well, I knew after fifteen years of attempting to eat right and checking the scale, it was time to learn how to do it RIGHT. Within five months, by applying all of the knowledge and guidance he afforded me, I did what I thought was impossible, and these were the results:

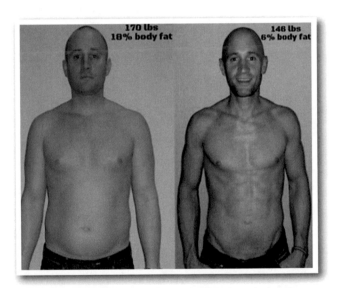

It was hard to believe, but I did what I had seen others do online and on television. I also did it exercising only one hour, 2-3 times a week. If I could have such great success, why can't you? This is not a gimmick and although I can't guarantee you will experience the same" before and after" results, it does work!

I am forever grateful to Chris Lentino for starting me on this journey. Now I would love to help you change your life as well. I have since earned my designation as a Fitness

Nutrition Specialist and continue to learn every day about the importance of diet in our lives. I wish I had a book like this one to guide me through my transformation. I wrote this book so that I could share all I know with you and give you the opportunity to succeed in living a healthier and leaner lifestyle!

Now It's Your Turn!

Congratulations on taking the first steps towards improving the health of your body and the quality of your life. The purpose of this book is to begin to help you understand what it takes to BURN FAT! Before you start though, it is important to consult with your physician whenever starting any exercise or diet plan. So please do so! The contents within have been selected to give you the most knowledge you need to complete your journey without overloading you with too much information.

In order to guide you in this eating plan, you will need to understand the principles required to do so. Specifically the main theme of this diet, as the title states is: **Macronutrients**. Since you will be doing most of the work, it helps to know the reasons for the decisions you are about to make. The skills and knowledge you will learn here will last a lifetime.

Throughout the book there are words, phrases and ideas we have attempted to clarify, but if you still don't understand a concept or idea please ask. This information is based on science and research about the topic of changing body composition. For your convenience and ease of read, most chapters are only one to two pages in length. I have also included a **"Take Away Message"** at the end of each chapter to summarize what you've just read.

The reality is that if you are committed to learning and adopting this methodology, you will experience a leaner and healthier lifestyle. Your body will thank you for it! But make no mistake, there is a decent amount of work initially. It's not for everyone! Personally, I had an amazing experience. I followed the program and strategies very closely. However, it still took over six months for me to totally understand all the information needed for me to succeed beyond the initial phases of this diet. For myself and the clients we work with, it is now a: MacroNutrient Lifestyle!

Included, is a complete three phase diet and exercise plan.

Take Away Message

There are specific principles and strategies to burning fat and getting lean and they are not secrets.   If you adhere to the ideas and principles in this book, you are sure to make visible changes in your appearance and most importantly, your health. Make no mistake, this program is initially difficult, and it is not for anyone who isn't totally committed to the process. Most people are overweight because they do not understand these concepts!

Follow the 70:20:10 Rule

Stop exercising for just a moment. It is NOT the way to lose weight and change body composition. Let's look closely at the 70:20:10 rule. This is a ratio you should adhere to when working toward changing body composition. When we think about losing weight or more specifically burning fat, most people resort to excessive and dangerous exercise routines, counting calories on the treadmill, and then putting all the wrong things in their bodies. **That is NOT the way!**

70%: The percentage that diet plays in burning fat. Eating food is a job and a blueprint used to manipulate the way your body handles energy. Success in changing body composition is largely the result of nutritional decisions alone!

20%: The percentage exercise plays in burning fat (and only the right exercise works! Hint: It's not Cardio) Building lean muscle through safe forms of resistance training is key in maximizing results. It's not spending 60 minutes on a treadmill or elliptical or in a Zumba class 6 days a week.

10%: The final component - Rest! For every day there must be a night, for every winter, a summer, for every inhale, an exhale, sunrise and sunset, life and death! It is the way of the universe. Rest is necessary for your body to repair and function at its best. Resting isn't being lazy; it's the time required for healing and energizing. Spend time resting!

Take Away Message

Mostly diet, not exercise, changes your body composition. Don't forget that all the work you do in a gym can easily be ruined with a few bites of the wrong food.

Other Diets

Knowing that diet is so important, why choose this one? Hopefully you will see that every diet is really just a macronutrient diet. The difference is that other diets attempt to make it so simple as to assume you don't have the capacity to learn about food. That's why you see things like counting points, or eating frozen, prepared meals. The thinking, understanding, and work is already done for you by someone else. Although these methods do create effective habits, and do work to help you lose weight in the short term, the problem is that these methods are unsustainable over time.

You need to face the fact that learning about your body and about the food you eat or feed your family, is necessary if you plan on maintaining healthy habits for the long haul. Knowing that diet has so many implications for preventing disease and feeling healthy, that it is worth the time and energy to start now.

Take Away Message

All kinds of diets work! That's because all diets come down to the same principles! What you will learn in this book are those principles!

Weight Loss vs. Body Composition (Body Fat %)

It is important to understand here that losing weight has no real value in and of itself, and it's not what you actually want anyway. Let's start by answering this question, "What is weight?"

What you weigh is really a combination of fat, muscle, bone, skin, water, undigested food in your GI tract, internal organs etc. Now, do you want it all to go away? NO, the reality is you want to keep and enhance the good stuff and get rid of the bad. This is what changing the composition of your body is all about. Getting lean. Not just losing weight.

Muscle and Lean Tissue = GOOD (we want more which may include weight gain)

Fat = BAD (we want less which will include weight loss)

Fat, by the way is perfectly handled by your body. When abundance is attained in the body, the nutrients are stored in little briefcases called fat cells which are in the periphery or the outer part of the body as well as surrounding organs. Fat acts as protection from the environment. It is also stored away to be used as energy for a later time when needed.

With the MacroNutrient Diet, we will be instituting strategies that will be aimed at burning fat and increasing lean tissue, not "losing weight." Losing weight will happen, but you may also gain muscle. That's why we need to use particular methods to measure progress. These methods include the use of a scale and either calipers or a tape measure.

Scale:

- Measures weight of entire body without regard to healthy or unhealthy tissue.

- Does not distinguish between fat and lean tissue.

- May not show a change if you gain muscle and lose fat.

Body Fat Measurements:

- Fat Caliper- Device used to pinch and measure amount of body fat in specific locations.

- Girth measurements - (Tape measure) used to measure girth at particular points of the body.

A scale is only used to measure the total weight of your body at one point in time and is **a poor way to measure progress or the current health and fat content of your body**. Therefore, your weight will be taken only for the purpose of figuring what percentage of you is lean and what percentage of you is fat. The following chart outlines normal body fat % for men and women at different ages.

MALE

Age	Very good	good	Average	Poor
10-14	<11%	11-16%	16.1-21%	>21.1%
15-19	<12%	12-17%	17.1-22%	>22.1%
20-29	<13%	13-18-%	18.1-23%	>23.1%
30-39	<14%	14-19%	19.1-24%	>24.1%
40-49	<15%	15-20%	20.1-25%	>25.1%
50-59	<16%	16-21%	21.1-26%	>26.1%
60-69	<17%	17-22%	22.1-27%	>27.1%
70-100	<18%	18-23%	23.1-28%	>28.1%

FEMALE

Age	Very good	Good	Average	Poor
10-14	<16%	16-21%	21.1-26%	>26.1%
15-19	<17%	17-22%	22.1-27%	>27.1%
20-29	<18%	18-23%	23.1-28%	>28.1%
30-39	<19%	19-24%	24.1-29%	>29.1%
40-49	<20%	20-25%	25.1-30%	>30.1%
50-59	<21%	21-26%	26.1-31%	>31.1%
60-69	<22%	22-27%	27.1-32%	>32.1%
70-100	<23%	23-28%	28.1-32%	>33.1%

Table 1

Take Away Message

Forget the phrase, "weight loss" and replace it with, "changing my body composition". After all, if you weigh more but look like an underwear model you won't care what you weigh and neither will anyone else.

NOTE: If you are going to weigh yourself, you must do it when you wake up in the morning, on the same scale, and in the same clothes. Expect a 1-2 pound error.

The Three Principles:

Quality, Quantity, Timing

These are the three principles of this diet. They are all intricately related and like a tripod, rely on one another to create changes in body composition. **Understand and memorize these three words!!!**

If you have ever bought a diamond, you know it's worth isn't just about the size: carats. The value is a combination of carats, color, cut, clarity, etc. A 10 carat diamond that is cloudy and dull has little value. One variable alone does not add value but when combined correctly with other qualities, the diamond becomes unique and valuable.

Diet also has a set of principles that all need to be combined correctly to get specific results. They are: the **QUALITY** of the food you eat, the **QUANTITY** of the food you eat, and the **TIMING** of the food you eat.

Principle #**1**: QUALITY: Approved food choices for carbs, fat, and protein are provided on pages 110 - 114. They are nutrient dense and healthy choices for burning fat on this plan. They are chosen as quality foods because of their rating on the Glycemic Index, their macro and micronutrient density, fiber levels and wholeness. You will need to choose quality foods to burn fat!

Principle #**2**: QUANTITY: The more food you eat, the more food energy you take in. Food energy that is not used, is stored as fat. You will have a "budget" you will need to stick to on this diet, or on any diet, for that matter.

Principle #**3**: TIMING: How often you eat or don't eat on any given day, plays a direct role in your ability to burn fat. You must eat every two to three hours but not more often. We will go into a bit more detail as to why this is, but for now, accept this as law! (Eat every 2-3 hours. NO more, no less)

Take Away Message

These are the foundational principles of this book and The MacroNutrient Diet. To do this program correctly, you must have these three factors working together. Or else you're just a 10 carat lump of coal! The program calls for six meals a day, eaten 2-3 hours apart, in the correct quantities, comprised of quality foods. End of story.

These are the principles of this diet!

INTRODUCTION

It all starts here! In order to begin to understand how to make long lasting changes in your nutrition and your body, you need to understand the basics about how the body works in the presence of food. You also need a basic understanding of macronutrients and the components of what is in the food you eat. Just telling you what to eat and when to eat it works in the short term. Unfortunately, it has no benefit if you plan on burning fat and keeping it off for good!

You must also come to know that macronutrients are the single foundation for any and all diets on the planet! Hence - The MacroNutrient Diet!

"Your body is merely a representation of your mind. Therefore, you can't change your body unless you change your mind!"

Food on Planet Earth

The purpose of eating food is simple: to nourish the body and to provide the raw materials to use as energy. **THAT'S IT!** For thousands of years it's been that way, and only in the last few centuries / decades has the focus changed. We now use food to create an experience either through size, flavor or texture.

Think about it, I want you to list the food choices you would have had 10,000 years ago? Here they are:

- wild game = fish and animals (meat / protein and fat)

- fruit and vegetables (fiber, carbohydrates, protein)

- Nuts (fat and protein)

And what about your choice of drinks?

- Water

- Milk (from another species of animal which to this day is a questionable practice)

- Water

- Water (get it?)

Nothing has changed. To make improvements in body composition and to get lean, we will be returning to a very simplistic set of choices including lean proteins, complex carbohydrates, fruits, vegetables, and the elimination of what I call "The Matrix." In the movie, "The Matrix" starring Keanu Reeves, there were really two worlds. These two worlds included the very simplistic "real" world and the modern day, "illusionary" world. "The Matrix" is the illusionary world that you are led to believe is real. With nutrition and food selection, "The Matrix" is just about any food that isn't on the list above, designed to create an experience. Some of these foods have nutritional value, but most of them are cleverly advertised and marketed to give you an "experience."

An example of this food is lightly sweetened , multi-grain cereal. According to the illusion it has little to no sugar and it apparently is loaded with wholesome grains. However when we look closer at the nutritional value, the grains are stripped of their nutrients and the ingredients are loaded with sugar. In "the Matrix" this appears to be a healthy food choice, but in the real world, this cereal is just an illusion of health to disguise empty calorie food.

Another example of this is the Wizard of Oz. A real grand wizard is he? On the outside he may be, but upon further investigation, he is just an old man behind a curtain with a microphone and a smoke machine.

Take Away Message

If you are going to change your body fat percentage, be prepared to reduce the number of food options available to you. You need to escape "The Matrix" and uncover "The Wizard of Oz". You will need to focus on changing your body not appeasing your mind.   By the way, appeasing your mind is only a fleeting, temporary thing. The next day you will have to do it again. Make choices towards healthy, fat burning nutrition and not because of the dreaded answer to everything, "it tastes good" or, "I like it".

Physiology Of Food And Burning Fat

In order to better understand the diet and nutritional choices we are about to make, you need a basic understanding of the digestive process.

Once food enters the mouth enzymes begin to break down the food, specifically carbohydrates. Food is chewed to break it up for swallowing and allow for easier digestion.

Once past the stomach and into the small intestine, absorption of specific nutrients begins. These nutrients are absorbed into the blood stream for transport. Once in the blood, certain chemicals are released by digestive organs. This includes Insulin as an example. The purpose is to collect all of the fat, protein and carbohydrate (glucose energy) from the absorbed food that is now in the bloodstream and deliver it to specific places in the body either for use or storage as fat.

This food energy is deposited and stored in the muscles and the rest in the liver where it sits waiting to be released and used as energy. (Although the liver functions to clean the blood, it is also the main player in your ability to get lean) All other excess food energy is stored as fat around organs and at the periphery under the skin throughout the body.

Protein is used to build muscle and it too, in excess, is stored as fat if not used. Fat is used to help absorb specific vitamins and minerals. It too will be stored as fat if not used. The rest of the contents of the food ingested like fiber, is passed as waste.

In abundance the body stores fat. In starvation, the body will destroy lean tissue and potentially store fat. Only with the correct balance can one be properly nourished while satisfying the requirements to burn fat.

Therefore, it is crucial for us to calculate your TDEE (Total Daily Energy Expenditure), so we know how many calories and grams of macronutrients your body needs in one day. From there, we create a deficit and ultimately start the process of changing body composition.

Take Away Message

Depending on the amount of food and the type eaten, the body will either use it as energy or store it as fat. Therefore, creating a diet based on quantity, quality, and timing, is the key to manipulating your body to burn fat rather than store it.

Insulin Response

I briefly described in the previous chapter that digestive organs release chemicals and hormones in order to deal with the food we eat. Because one of these hormones is extremely important in either burning or storing fat, I want to go into a bit more detail. It's known as insulin.

Insulin is like the fat storage hormone. Depending on the food we decide to eat and the quantity of that food, our body determines the amount of insulin to release. The more insulin we release, the more sugar is extracted from our blood stream and brought to the cells of our body. This makes it more likely that we overload our energy needs. This excess food energy is then stored as fat.

The right macronutrients: complex carbs, lean protein, and healthy fats stabilize your insulin levels. That's why we provide a list of approved items on pages 110 - 114 in this book. Choosing these types of foods is paramount to your success!

Wouldn't it be nice to know if a food were going to cause an insulin response before you even eat it? Well, it just so happens you can. It's called the Glycemic Index and Glycemic Load of a particular food. This concept is explained in the next chapter in this book!

Take Away Message

A high Insulin response causes fat storage. The food we eat determines that insulin response. Therefore, choosing foods that limit your insulin response will promote fat burning and improve your body composition. Knowing the Glycemic Index and Glycemic Load of your food choices helps you manage this insulin response.

Glycemic Index And Glycemic Load

Managing Your Insulin Response

There is so much talk about Glycemic Index and believe it or not, there is still some conflicting evidence about this idea. But, for now, accept it as law! Remember, we learned that the insulin response is caused by the quality and quantity of the food you eat. Therefore keeping a low and steady insulin response is crucial. The higher the Glycemic Load and Index of a food, the higher the insulin response and the more fat storage. Made famous by the South Beach diet, the idea of leveling your Glycemic Index has huge implications with body fat.

The Glycemic Index (GI) ranks specific carbohydrates from zero to 100, based on the rate in which they affect your insulin response. A GI of 1 to 55 is low, 56 to 69 is medium, and 70 to 100 is high – these high-ranking foods should be limited or even eliminated. (i.e. a slice of white bread is equal to a GI of 100)

Just when you started to get a handle on the Glycemic Index (GI) of foods, there's another value to grasp – Glycemic Load (GL). Glycemic Load measures the blood-sugar-raising power per serving of food. Simply stated, it relates to the quantity of the food you eat. So you need to consider the Glycemic Index of the food compounded by the amount of that food you ingest in order to get the Glycemic Load. A Glycemic Load of 10 or less is low, 11 to 19 is medium, 20 or more is high. If you add up the Glycemic Load amounts for your entire day, a total GL amount of 80 or less is considered low. Your daily GL shouldn't exceed 120.

Both measurements are useful. **Glycemic Load implies amount, while Glycemic Index implies the likelihood of a more intense insulin response.** (not exactly, but close enough for your understanding at this time) The lower each number, the less it affects insulin levels, and the less likely you are to store fat.

Food	GI	GL
1 medium apple	38	6
1 small banana	47	8
10 baby carrots	35	2
1 medium baked potato with skin	76	23
1 medium orange	42	5
1 medium pear	38	4
1 cup white rice	64	23
1 cup brown rice	55	18
1 cup regular pasta	44	18
1 cup whole wheat pasta	37	14
1 cup skim milk	32	4
1 oz. cashews	22	2

Table 2

The MacroNutrient Diet

Go to www.NutritionData.com, enter the name of a food, and it will tell you the GLYCEMIC LOAD.

Go to www.Montignac.com, enter the name of a food, and it'll tell you the GLYCEMIC INDEX.

Take Away Message

Don't worry so much about Glycemic Load except that the larger the portion, the greater the insulin response. Instead, be thinking about choosing low glycemic foods. By the way, any food with a Glycemic Index rated below 25 causes little or no insulin response. Cherries, for example, have a GI of 22. So, unless you eat way too many, no insulin response! It's a better choice for burning fat than an orange, or a pear.

Food As A Blueprint

As you can see in the last few sections, food is really a set of instructions to tell the body how to respond. These "messages", in turn, create body composition. The blueprint for a home is just a set of instructions that shows what the house will look like when built. Food is that blueprint! Simply stated, you will use food (instructions) to either store fat or burn fat!

What most people refuse to believe, is that exercise is **NOT** the key to looking the way you want. Being lean comes from particular diet habits! Looking lean and healthy comes from **DIET!** Exercise is used to build lean tissue like muscle and expend energy stores, but without diet, exercise usually leads to the potential for injury.

We use fat, protein, and carbohydrates in food, in a similar way to the wood, metal and cement used in building a house. They are the raw materials and the blueprint to manipulate the normal processes of the body. This process is what makes you a fat burning machine!

Take Away Message

Food is merely a blueprint and the raw materials to determine your body composition: basically, what your "home" (your body) will look and feel like. Which home would you rather live in?

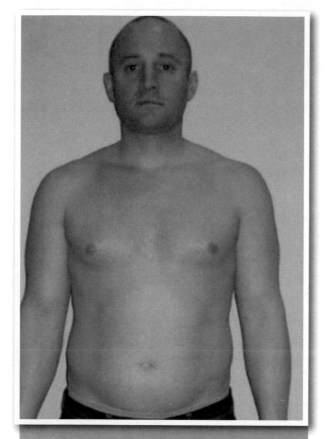

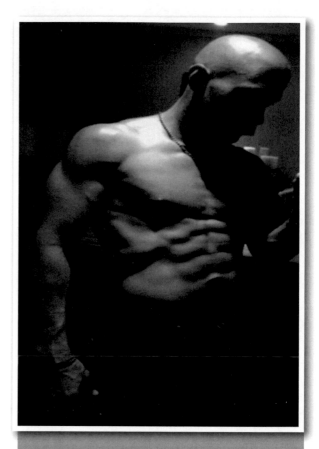

Eating poor quality foods at the wrong times and in the wrong quantities without any macronutrient accountability is the blueprint for this person. Poor Quality, Quantity & Timing!	**vs.**	Eating nutrient dense foods, at the right times, and in the right quantities with macronutrient accountability is the blueprint for this person. **Good Quality, Quantity, & Timing!**

Again, it all comes back to the three principles: Quality, Quantity and Timing. The choice is yours. This book is the guide. Now, let's build a new blueprint and a new body for you!

Supplementation

The Dietary Guidelines for Americans make it clear that your nutritional needs should be met primarily through your diet. For some people, however, supplements may be a useful way to get nutrients they might otherwise be lacking. But before you go shopping for supplements, get the facts on what they will and won't do for you.

Supplements vs. Whole Foods

Supplements aren't intended to be a food substitute because they can't replicate all of the nutrients and benefits of whole foods, such as fruits and vegetables. So depending on your situation and your eating habits, dietary supplements may not be worth the expense.

Whole foods offer three main benefits over dietary supplements:

- **Greater nutrition.** Whole foods are complex and contain a variety of the micronutrients your body needs – not just one. An orange, for example, provides vitamin C plus some beta carotene, calcium and other nutrients. A vitamin C supplement lacks these other micronutrients.

- **Essential fiber.** Whole foods, such as whole grains, fruits, vegetables and legumes, provide dietary fiber. Most high-fiber foods are also packed with other essential nutrients. Fiber, as part of a healthy diet, can help prevent certain diseases, such as type 2 diabetes and heart disease, and it can also help manage constipation.

- **Protective substances.** Whole foods contain other substances important for good health. Fruits and vegetables, for example, contain naturally occurring substances called phytochemicals, which may help protect you against cancer, heart disease, diabetes and high blood pressure. Many are also good sources of antioxidants – substances that slow down oxidation, a natural process that leads to cell and tissue damage.

With that being said, for this particular eating plan, it may be difficult to maintain 6 -7 meals completely with whole foods. Personally 3 of my 6-7 meals are supplemented with protein shakes or Quest Bars containing particular macronutrients.

I have included the web address of my Amazon store here. There you will find approved supplemental products for both whey, casein, and plant based protein powders, bars, shaker bottles, complex carbs, etc. It's through Amazon so orders over $35 usually ship free but feel free to shop around for your own products. Whatever you do, avoid products that contain saturated fats, and sugars. Here is the link:

http://astore.amazon.com/macronutrientdiet-20

Take Away Message

It's always better to get your macros from food, but let's face it, who has the time? Making 2-3 meals throughout the day a supplement makes it easy to hit your macronutrient targets, and a quick and easy way to make sure you don't go without eating. There are tons of supplements out there and most of them are loaded with all the wrong stuff. Not all protein powders are created equally. (Try to keep protein powders carbohydrate free) Food is a job, just get your macros and move on!!!

PRINCIPLE #1: QUALITY

The quality of the food you eat is one of the three main principles of the MacroNutrient Diet and is crucial to your success. Quality foods are chosen because of their rating on the Glycemic Index, their macro and micronutrient density, fiber levels, and wholeness. You will need to choose quality foods to burn fat!

NOTE: Nutritional information is now more readily available than ever. We recommend that you use these tools to track and learn about the macronutrients you eat. Over time you will get better at recognizing nutritionally appropriate foods. Our #1 recommended nutritional data resource is the app, "Fooducate." It has a scanner, shopping list feature, and the ability to compare products!

#1 CHOICE: iphone app: Fooducate

www.nutritiondata.self.com

www.caloriecount.com

http://ndb.nal.usda.gov/

Macronutrients - This is the Foundation!

The energy (a.k.a. calories) in the food we eat comes from three macronutrients: proteins, fats, and carbohydrates. Macro means large, and these nutrients are needed in large quantities to sustain our growth, metabolism, and other bodily functions. Our bodies require other nutrients, too, including vitamins and minerals. However, these nutrients are required in smaller quantities and are therefore called micronutrients. While critical to our health, micronutrients do not provide us with significant energy.

Protein

(A list of acceptable sources of Proteins are listed on page 113)

Protein is the main component of our lean body mass and it's used to rebuild tissues in the body. By eating adequate protein you will be able to increase your lean muscle mass (via the stimulus of resistance training), increase metabolism (via a number of mechanisms), and signal hormone production that reduces the storage of body fat.

There are twenty different amino acids, and all of them must be present in order for our bodies to build, maintain, and repair themselves. Nine of the 20 amino acids are considered essential because they cannot be manufactured by your body; they must come from food sources. Proteins that contain all twenty amino acids are called complete proteins, and they are found in animal sources: meat, poultry, fish, and dairy (eggs and milk products). Proteins that come from plant sources are considered incomplete because they do not contain all twenty amino acids, though you can combine different plant sources to obtain all of them.

It is a common misconception that you must eat animal products in order to supply your body with enough protein. In fact, if you compare meat and dairy to dark green vegetables, soybeans, and other plant sources, you will find that the plant foods often contain more protein, based on an equal number of calories, than their animal counterparts.

Fat

(A list of acceptable sources of fats are listed on page 114)

Fat, like protein, is necessary to maintain a healthy body. It is a vital component for building body tissue and cells, and it aids in the absorption of some vitamins and other nutrients. And just as there are essential amino acids, there are essential fatty acids which must come from food sources.

Just like all macronutrients, there are good fat sources and bad fat sources. Many people eat too much of the bad fats, but also eat too little of the good fats required for optimal health. The **bad fats include:** saturated fats and trans fats. The **good fats include:** unsaturated fats (monounsaturated and polyunsaturated) and the essential fatty acids (primarily omega-3 and omega-6). Cholesterol is a fat found only in animal products. It is already produced in the body at the levels needed so added cholesterol is on the watch list.

It's not just the fat we eat that can become fat on our bodies. **Any macronutrient not immediately needed by our bodies is stored in our energy reserves of body fat.** When needed, it can be broken down and used for energy. Though all too often it is just left to sit there.

Carbohydrates

(A list of acceptable sources of carbohydrates are listed on page 111 - 112)

Carbohydrates are chains of small, simple sugars, and are the **body's main source of fuel.** They are broken down and enter the bloodstream as glucose. Excess glucose is stored in the form of glycogen in the liver and, in limited quantities, the muscles. Carbohydrates are not your enemy, simple carbohydrates are!

- Simple carbohydrates are small molecules. Because of their size, they can be metabolized quickly and therefore provide the quickest source of energy. They include the various forms of sugar, such as sucrose (table sugar), fructose (fruit sugar), and lactose (dairy sugar) to name a few. Remember, sugar is sugar is sugar regardless of where it comes from so avoiding it is crucial to burning fat.

- Complex carbohydrates are larger molecules. Because they are larger, it takes longer for your body to metabolize them to provide energy. They include starch, glycogen, and cellulose, and are found in vegetables and unrefined whole grains. Complex carbohydrates are also excellent sources of fiber.

- Fiber is a form of carbohydrate that our bodies cannot digest. It is not only important for health, but is a significant factor in weight loss and changing body composition. (Of the carbohydrates listed on food labels, fiber is good and sugar is bad)

Alcohol

(Should be eliminated all together in order to maximize results)

First: Alcohol is also a substance that must be dealt with by the body. Unfortunately, when ingested, it is primarily sugar. It is used as a primary energy source. In other words, your body must process alcohol before any other macronutrients. This process increases the chances that other macros will be stored as fat.

Second: Alcohol must be metabolized by the liver. Occupying your liver with alcohol prevents the efficiency of burning fat.

Third: I don't know about you, but drinking alcohol without eating or snacking is difficult and certainly leads you into temptation.

As you will learn a few chapters from here, each gram of macronutrient has a caloric equivalent. Fat has 9 calories per gram, carbs have 4 calories per gram, protein has 4 calories per gram and alcohol has: 7 calories per gram! Only 2 calories less than fat!

Last, drinking usually goes on for several hours so ingesting sugar for long periods of time is a sure way to create an insulin reaction and store fat. For the purposes of this eating plan alcohol should be avoided, and now you know the reason!

Macronutrient Accountability

For The MacroNutrient Diet and potentially for your lifetime, you are responsible to track and be accountable for the quality, quantity, and timing of the macronutrients you eat each day.

Take Away Message

Understanding macronutrients is crucial to succeeding on this journey. After all, we named the diet after them. They are life and they are the foundation of this program. Lean proteins, healthy fats, and complex carbohydrates in particular amounts and at particular times are the blueprint for fat loss.

Micronutrients

Micronutrients are what are commonly referred to as "vitamins and minerals." Micronutrients include such minerals as fluoride, selenium, sodium, iodine, copper and zinc. They also include vitamins such as vitamin C, A, D, E and K, as well as the B-complex vitamins.

As mentioned, micronutrients are different from the macronutrients(protein, carbohydrates and fat). Micronutrients are called "micro"-nutrients because your body needs only very small quantities of them for survival. However, if your body doesn't get the small quantities of micronutrients that it needs, serious health problems can result.

Take Away Message

Micronutrients are crucial in the right amounts and assist in the many functions of your diet. Without getting into too much detail here, these are found in the foods you eat and can be supplemented with multi-vitamins. Please consult with your physician about the appropriate supplementation plan.

Sugar

The New Fat

Sugar is the simplest form of one of your macronutrients: carbohydrates. It is important to single this one out because of how dangerous and damaging it is to your body and the body's ability to burn fat.

Decades ago, the fat content in our foods was said to be the cause of many human illnesses like coronary artery disease for example. It turns out that was only partially right. In response, companies have replaced the fat in our foods with sugar to preserve and enhance flavor. Unfortunately, simple sugar is just a trigger for an insulin response. As you just learned, this is the blueprint for storing fat!

Sugar is already found naturally in foods. Fortunately, when ingested with the fiber and selected from the fruit list in the "list of acceptable carbohydrates" (pages 111 - 112) the effects on the body are far less damaging.

Sugar is energy. Remember it is taken up in the blood stream by insulin and delivered to the cells of the body. When needed during exercise, sugar (glucose once in the body) helps sustain energy levels. That's why you see professional athletes with little body fat drinking Gatorade. For people who are extremely athletic for long periods of time, quick sugar is needed for replenishing energy stores. For most of us however, this isn't the case. That's why drinking a Gatorade with lunch, delivers sugar to cells that don't need it.

It would be like trying to fill a gas tank that was already full. The excess would just spill over. In your body when your cells are already full, the excess is stored as fat.

It's one thing for food to have sugar, it's another thing if the food has "added" sugar. For example fruit has natural sugar in it called fructose. Milk has a natural sugar called lactose. Added sugar would be like rolling a strawberry in a coating of table sugar. The fructose from the strawberry combined with the added sugar is NO GOOD! Check the ingredients on the label. (There is a section about label reading on page 37)

The following is a list of the many ways companies list sugar in disguise:

> Agave Nectar, Barley Malt Syrup, Beet Sugar, Brown Rice Syrup, Brown Sugar, Cane Crystals (or, even better, "cane juice crystals"), Cane Sugar, Coconut Sugar, or Coconut Palm Sugar, Corn sweetener, Corn syrup, or corn syrup solids, Dehydrated Cane Juice, Dextrin, Dextrose, Evaporated Cane Juice, Fructose, Fruit juice concentrate, Glucose, High-fructose corn syrup, Honey, Invert sugar, Lactose, Maltodextrin, Malt syrup, Maltose, Maple syrup, Molasses, Palm Sugar, Raw sugar, Rice Syrup, Saccharose, Sorghum or sorghum syrup, Sucrose, Syrup, Treacle, Turbinado Sugar, Xylose

Take Away Message

Sugar, on this diet is a NO NO! Check the labels of the foods you eat for macronutrients and under the carbohydrate section, check sugar. Be prepared to be shocked at how many foods have sugar, and in large quantities. For example even some of the best, healthiest, plain yogurts have over 8 grams of sugar. On this plan, it is suggested that less than 15-20 grams of your carbohydrates come from sugar. As you will learn, all carbohydrates need to be complex!

Finally, on page 129, there is an article by Dr. Dwight Lundell, a cardiovascular surgeon. Read it now or when you get to it, but make sure you read it!!! If you don't believe me that sugar is an enemy to becoming lean and healthy, you soon will!

4 grams of sugar = 1 teaspoon

Nutrient Dense Vs. Empty Calorie Food

Simply put, nutrient dense foods are those with the most amount of macronutrients and micronutrients and the least amount of calories. Empty calorie foods have low amounts of quality macronutrients and micronutrients with the same or higher amounts of calories. The major disadvantage of frequently consuming empty-calorie foods is that energy intake can easily exceed energy requirements without any nourishment to the body. If not used for physical activity, the extra calories are stored in the body as fat, and over time, result in weight gain and obesity.

Most empty-calorie foods are highly processed foods that contain added fat and sugar. Examples include baked products such as cakes, cookies, pies and pastries as well as puddings, doughnuts, fries, jams, syrups, jelly, sweetened fruit drinks, fried burgers and ice cream. Empty-calorie foods also make up most of the long shelf life foods and beverages sold in vending machines such as chips, salted snacks, candy, soda, energy and sports drinks. Although empty-calorie foods are cheaper and more readily available than nutrient-dense foods, habitual consumption of these foods can have a negative effect on health and will cause you to store fat. **(On The MacroNutrient Diet, you cannot eat these and expect results!)**

Eating a healthy, balanced diet of nutrient-dense foods provides many nutrients that are required to maintain health. Planning meals that include fruits, vegetables, whole grains, nuts, beans, seeds, turkey, chicken, fish and lean cuts of meats is essential. These foods provide fewer calories but are excellent sources of nutrients such as the B-vitamins, vitamins A, C, D and E, protein, calcium, iron, potassium, zinc, fiber and monounsaturated fatty acids. Fruits and vegetables also contain phytochemicals that may help reduce the incidence of heart disease, diabetes and cancer. They also promote a leaner you!

Let's say you are a calorie counter and you need roughly 150 calories. As an extreme example, you can eat 7 Swedish fish candies or 1 cup of cubed yams. Take a look:

Comparison of Empty Calorie Food(Swedish fish candy) vs. Nutrient Dense Food (Yams)							
Food item	**Serving Size**	**Calories**	**Fat**	**Protein**	**Carbs**	**Fiber**	**Sugar**
Swedish Fish Candy	7 pieces 40g	140	0g	0g	35g	0g	28g
Yams (cubed)	1 cup 136g	158	<1g	2g	37.4g	5.3g	<1g

Table 3

For almost the same calories, you would be eating more than three times the amount of yams as Swedish fish while getting fiber, healthy fat, potassium, protein vitamins, and almost no sugar. By the way, one teaspoon of granulated sugar equals 4 grams of sugar. To put it another way, the 28 **grams** of sugar in the Swedish fish is equal to about 7 teaspoons of granulated sugar.

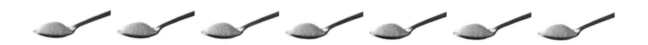

Yam: Nutrient dense   **Swedish Fish:** Empty calorie

Take Away Message

To burn fat on The MacroNutrient Diet, you must eat nutrient dense foods only!!!

Reading Food Labels

Location of Information Regarding Your Macronutrients

In order to stop counting calories and start hitting your macronutrient targets for the day you will need to constantly be looking at labels. Here is a quick overview. Avoid sugar!! It's the new FAT!

You have permission to stop reading the front of all food packages. That's the area where marketers try to convince you to choose their product over the others that are sitting next to it on the shelf. The real information you're looking for is on the nutrition panel side.

When you choose packaged food, always turn the package over and read the Nutrition Facts panel. This panel, together with the ingredient list below it, tells you what is actually in the product. Here is the order of label reading:

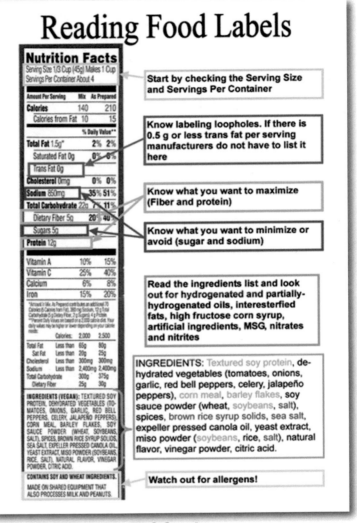

Table 4

1. Check the serving size- you may need to double the macronutrients and calories if you exceed the amount listed (i.e. in this label the serving size is 1/3 cup and the bag contains 4 servings. That means if you use the whole bag you will have to multiply the macronutrients and calories by 4)

2. Although I usually look at calories, they don't mean much. What's more important are the macronutrients. After all the calories are calculated according to the macros anyway.

3. Look at the amount of fat to make sure it fits your macro goals for the day. Trans fat and saturated are bad while mono and polyunsaturated fats are good. *** This is one of your three macronutrients!**

4. Look at the number of carbohydrates. More importantly look at the breakdown of them. High fiber is good, while sugar content is bad. Unfortunately, this section of the label does not distinguish between the natural sugar found in a food and added sugar. It is all combined in the sugar contents so reading the ingredients allows you to see if they added sugar on top of what is already in the food. Remember, limit sugar to between 15-20 grams a day! *** This is the second of your three macronutrients!**

5. Look at the amount of protein and make sure it too fits into your macronutrient equation for the day. *** This is the final of your three macronutrients!**

6. Finally, look at the ingredients list. The ingredients in the food appear in order of greatest content to least content so the first 1-3 ingredients are usually the most important. Be on the lookout for the hidden sugars and refined flour.

Take Away Message:

The back of the package is where it's at! Look for fat, carbs, protein, fiber (your macros) and make sure they are consistent with the macros you need for the day. Finally, check the ingredients and avoid sugar! The best iPhone app to use is "Fooducate"

Bread: You Already Know The Answer To This! Don't Bother!

Seriously, bread is a tricky subject because there is so much bad information out there and marketing companies have done an amazing job of fooling you to believe something is healthy.

Bread is a carbohydrate and the only way it can be good for you is if it's whole grain bread, and whole grain bread only! The ingredients have to say Whole Grain! Don't read the front of the package. You have to look at the ingredients!

Below is a chart to help you identify the right bread:

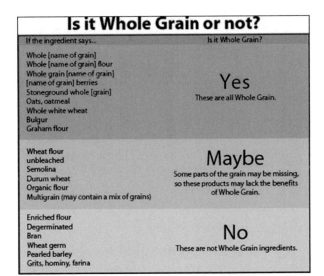

Is it Whole Grain or not?

If the ingredient says...	Is it Whole Grain?
Whole [name of grain] Whole [name of grain] flour Whole grain [name of grain] [name of grain] berries Stoneground whole [grain] Oats, oatmeal Whole white wheat Bulgur Graham flour	**Yes** These are all Whole Grain.
Wheat flour unbleached Semolina Durum wheat Organic flour Multigrain (may contain a mix of grains)	**Maybe** Some parts of the grain may be missing, so these products may lack the benefits of Whole Grain.
Enriched flour Degerminated Bran Wheat germ Pearled barley Grits, hominy, farina	**No** These are not Whole Grain ingredients.

Below is an example of Ezekiel bread (GOOD):

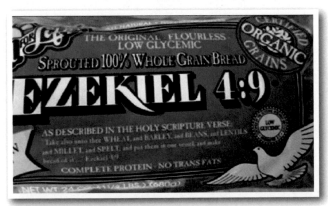

INGREDIENTS: ORG SPROUTED WHEAT, ORG SPROUTED BARLEY, ORG SPROUTED MILLET, ORG MALTED BARLEY, ORG SPROUTED LENTILS, ORG SPROUTED SOYBEANS, ORG SPROUTED SPELT, FILTERED WATER, FRESH YEAST, SEA SALT.

Below is an example of bad ingredients. Notice the first ingredient isn't whole grain. Also notice all the sugar and high fructose corn syrup (BAD):

MADE FROM: UNBROMATED UNBLEACHED ENRICHED WHEAT FLOUR (FLOUR, NIACIN, REDUCED IRON, THIAMINE MONONITRATE [VITAMIN B1], RIBOFLAVIN [VITAMIN B2], FOLIC ACID), WATER, YEAST, SOYBEAN OIL, HIGH FRUCTOSE CORN SYRUP, CONTAINS 2 PERCENT OR LESS OF: SALT, NATURAL FLAVORS, WHEAT GLUTEN, CALCIUM PROPIONATE AND SORBIC ACID TO RETARD SPOILAGE, LOWER SODIUM NATURAL SEA SALT, SUGAR, SESAME SEEDS, WHEAT FLOUR, MONOGLYCERIDES, DEXTROSE, MALTED WHEAT FLOUR, DATEM (DOUGH CONDITIONER), ENZYMES, CALCIUM CARBONATE, MALTED BARLEY FLOUR, NONFAT MILK*, DEHYDRATED SOUR DOUGH, GUAR GUM, CORNSTARCH, RYE FLOUR.
ADDS A TRIVIAL AMOUNT OF CHOLESTEROL.

Take Away Message:

Bread is usually a bad choice unless it fits your macros and it is the right kind. There are some good ones out there but they are not easy to find. Read your labels and ingredients and make the right choice! We believe in Ezekiel bread. If you can't find it at the grocery store, we have a link for it on our Amazon site: http://astore.amazon.com/ macronutrientdiet-20

The Organic Food Mistake

Organic food is certainly the best option when it comes to food because it means you are eating food that has been grown and raised as it was for hundreds of years. Unfortunately, people assume organic means it may be more likely to help you lose weight or get lean and that is a mistake! For example there is organic sugar. It is still a simple carbohydrate, it still has 4 calories per gram, and in large quantities still causes your body to store fat! Therefore, for this book, I want you to understand that organic really just means clean. You can eat all the wrong organic food, in all the wrong quantities and at all the wrong times and never lose a pound of fat. But, it is clean eating!

Organically grown produce generally costs more, but for the money, does organic food provide better macronutrients?

The answer is NO. Let me help you understand this a bit better. The word "organic" refers to the way farmers grow and process agricultural products, such as fruits, vegetables, grains, dairy products and meat. To simplify, farmers who grow organic produce, do it the clean, old fashioned way!

Here are some key differences between conventional farming and organic farming:

Conventional	Organic
Apply chemical fertilizers to promote plant growth.	Apply natural fertilizers, such as manure or compost, to feed soil and plants.
Spray synthetic insecticides to reduce pests and disease.	Spray pesticides from natural sources; use beneficial insects and birds, mating disruption or traps to reduce pests and disease.
Use synthetic herbicides to manage weeds.	Use environmentally-generated plant-killing compounds; rotate crops, till, hand weed or mulch to manage weeds.
Give animals antibiotics, growth hormones and medications to prevent disease and spur growth.	Give animals organic feed and allow them access to the outdoors. Use preventive measures — such as rotational grazing, a balanced diet and clean housing — to help minimize disease.

Table 5

But what if it says "Natural"

"Natural" and "Organic" are not interchangeable terms. You may see "natural" and other terms such as "all natural," "free-range" or "hormone-free" on food labels. These descriptions must be truthful, but don't confuse them with the term "organic." Only foods that are grown and processed according to USDA organic standards can be labeled organic.

More importantly, how does this all affect your macronutrients?

A recent study examined the past 50 years' worth of scientific articles about the macronutrient and micronutrient content of organic and conventional foods. **The researchers concluded that macronutrient and micronutrient content between organically and conventionally produced foods are relatively the same!**

Take Away Message:

There are no macronutrient differences between organic and conventional foods. So don't make the mistake that organically grown foods change anything about your macronutrient accountability. An organic burrito with all the wrong protein, carbs and fat will not help you get lean in the least bit. Although I would argue choosing organic food is overall better for you, macronutrient wise, it is the same thing only cleaner, and more costly. Organic just means CLEAN!

PRINCIPLE #2: QUANTITY

The quantity of the food you eat is the second of the three main principles of the MacroNutrient Diet. The more food you eat, the more food energy you take in. Food energy that is not used, is stored as fat. You will have a "budget" or a "quantity" of grams of macronutrients that you will need to adhere to every day. This is true for this diet and on any other diet for that matter.

Don't Count Calories Count Macronutrients!

A calorie is a unit of energy. In nutrition and everyday language, calories refer to energy consumption through eating and drinking and energy usage through physical activity. For example, an apple may have 80 calories, while a 1 mile walk may use up about 100 calories.

Most people associate calories just with food and drink, but **anything that contains energy has calories**. One ton of coal contains the equivalent in energy of 7,004,684,512 calories.

The human body needs calories (energy) to survive. Without energy our cells would die, our hearts and lungs would stop, and we would die. We acquire this energy from food and water. If we consume just the number of calories our body needs each day, every day, we will probably enjoy happy and healthy lives. If our calorie consumption is low or high, we will either burn or store fat.

The number of calories foods contain tells us how much potential energy they posses. Below are the caloric values of the three macronutrients we eat and are absolutes: (Memorize this. It will never, ever change.)

- 1 gram of **carbohydrates** contain....................**4 calories**

- 1 gram of **protein** contains.............................**4 calories**

- 1 gram of **fat** contains.....................................**9 calories**

- 1 gram of **alcohol** contains..............................**7 calories**

- **Sugar Alcohols contain**...............................**2.5 Calories (about half the amount of regular sugar)**

Let's look at an example of why we no longer need to count calories, but do need to focus on the macronutrients in our food. We will simply use the conversions above to do this from now on. If a protein shake has 10 grams of carbs, 20 grams of protein and 5 grams of fat, then we have all the info we need.

10 grams of carbs x 4 calories = 40 calories

20 grams of protein x 4 calories = 80 calories

5 grams of fat x 9 calories = 45 calories

Therefore, this shake has roughly 165 calories. Because these equivalents are always the same, when we give you the amount of protein, carbs, and fat you need in a day, if you stick to the grams allowed you will always be within your calorie range. So, don't count calories, count macros!

Now let's consider this. In the example above, let's say the calories are lumps of coal that need to either be burned or stored. You now have 165 lumps of coal you must use as energy and if not you will store them as FAT. The fat on your legs, stomach, and arms are just merely excess coal that your body didn't burn. This is why people think they need to being doing tons of cardio to burn fat, but they are wrong. Using food as a blueprint combined with the right kind of exercise is the way to burn fat and change your body composition.

Take Away Message

Stop counting calories and begin to take note of the grams of macronutrients in the foods you eat by looking at serving size and the macro amounts on the label. When you hit your macronutrient targets for the day you will be right on with your calories.

It's All Just A Math Equation: 2+2 +1 =5 will always be true!

It may seem hard to believe that changing your body composition is as easy as 2+2+1=5, but it really is. Most people have put way too much emotion and mental anguish into their weight and body image, but your weight, body composition and how you look in a bathing suit is simply a representation of your past behavior. In this very moment you are just a creation of all the diet and exercise choices you have made to this point in time. If you want to change that in the future, just change your current behavior. This book is the road map.

Most people attempt to eat healthy to lose weight but don't realize that the amount and type of food they eat just doesn't add up to the results they want. **This is precisely why most people convince themselves they are eating "healthy" and maybe they are, but not eating to burn fat!** Let me show you.

If I calculate your current body fat percentage, factor in age and exercise level, I can get your *TDEE (Total Daily Energy Expenditure: Total calories you need to maintain your current situation)* Based on that number I can create a deficit of calories. Because we already learned how many calories are in 1 gram of carbs,(4) protein(4), and fat(9), I can work backwards and tell you the number of grams of each macronutrient you will need to ingest each day to begin to change your body composition.

Therefore by the end of the day if you take in the number of grams of each and they add up to the totals of your target, you will end up with the correct number of calories at the end of the day. You will be nourished and your body will change. **The following are not actual amounts for your macros, but as an example, 2(protein)+2(carb)+1(fat)=5.** It's just math. No emotion, no guessing!! Your job is to make sure at the end of the day you don't add **5+1+1 (=7)** and expect 5 to be the answer. This error is a very common problem with those of you trying to burn fat.

Let's look at a real life, side by side comparison of a single meal that appears to be very similar at face value. Person A and person B are both drinking protein shakes. Both use the same amount of each ingredients to keep the size of the shakes identical. Let's say the macronutrient intake for this meal needs to be 10g of carbs, 30g of protein, and 5g of fat.

Food item	Serving Size	Calories	Fat	Protein	Carbs	Fiber	Sugar
Comparison of 2 similar but very different Kale shakes with blueberries and almond milk							
Person A: Kale, blueberries, (unsweetened, vanilla almond milk), P90X post-workout powder	1 shake 8oz	240	4g	14g	54.5g	5g	36g
Person B: Kale, blueberries, (sweetened, vanilla almond milk), Isopure vanilla protein powder	1 shake 8oz	200	3g	29g	8.5g	4g	4g

Table 6

As you can see according to the macros they need, person B almost hits each one right on. Person A has chosen the **same shake recipe, but the wrong ingredients (Quality.)** The macros simply don't add up. They both think they are drinking 2+2+1=5 but person A is drinking 5+1+1= 5? I don't think so. That equals 7.

Person A:

-The carbohydrates double what is needed

-The protein is only half of what was needed

-The Sugar is a staggering 36 grams

 (almost 2 days worth of sugar in 1 meal!)

Person B:

On target with macros and very little sugar

Aren't they drinking the same shake? Not according to the macronutrient values of fat, carbohydrates, and protein. Not according to the macro math. Same looking drink, completely different math equation. Person B is on target to get lean and Person A is drinking a blueprint for fat storage. Get it? It's just math!

One More Equation to Prove it's all just a simple formula

There is an equation in physics that states the following:

Power = Work over Time

So, what does that have to do with getting lean?

Getting lean (the product) = **The right diet plan**(variable 1) over a **period of time**(variable 2)

If you are not lean (the product), and you know you can't control time (variable 2), then there is only one thing to do. The Right work (variable 1) or the right diet plan (This one! Another cheap plug). It's that simple. It's just physics. You have a physical issue so your body has to abide by the physical laws of the planet.

Take Away Message

Once your body composition is measured and you know your macronutrient math equation, all you have to do is eat the right foods at the right times in the right amounts so at the end of the day your equation adds up. Your body will change!! It's all just a math equation. No emotion. Just science! Trust it! Failure to accept this is like failing to accept the earth is round.

PRINCIPLE #3: TIMING

The timing of the food you eat is the last of the three main principles of the MacroNutrient Diet. Eating small meals throughout the day is the blueprint for burning fat. We are well aware that this is nothing new in the diet world and that's for good reason, because it works. On this diet you must time your meals to succeed!

Starvation (Skipping Meals)

It's hard to explain to someone who has nearly or fully starved himself/herself for a few days that what he/she is doing isn't effective. The proof is right there on the scale, right? Two pounds, five pounds, ten pounds flushed from their bodies like that, simply by not eating.

Wrong. Losing real weight from starving is physically impossible. Your body absolutely cannot lose that much weight in a week. It's not because you weren't working hard enough, or didn't starve for long enough. The truth is that you cant lose weight and keep it off by starving.

Here's what happens when your body is starved of macronutrients:

Your body realizes that it needs energy to continue to function. All of this requires a power source, and it has to get it from somewhere. When you don't give your body the energy it needs from food, it cannibalizes itself as an energy source. The prime directive of the body is that it must have energy at any cost.

Although your body will begin to use fat stores, the protein in your muscles is the only other energy source a starving person has; since you aren't eating, your body will begin to destroy muscle cells to release that protein to convert it into energy. Muscles are about 70% water, so when a muscle cell is destroyed, that water is released and eventually excreted. That's your weight loss.

Your body didn't convert any lumpy fat into lean muscle. It didn't begin to use fat as an energy source. It didn't just magically get rid of three or four pounds of pure fat. It's going to keep you alive at any cost, and that means burning up the muscle and using that energy to power you. Guess what? You've just increased your body fat percentage. Fat weighs less than muscle and takes up more space. Therefore, you might even look bigger than before.

You've also lowered your metabolism. Muscle is metabolically active tissue, so the more muscle you have, the higher your metabolic rate. The next bite of food you take, your body will use less efficiently and will hold on to much longer by converting it into fat and storing it for the long perceived famine ahead.

Starving is not an effective weight loss tool. Not just because you shouldn't starve yourself, not just because of the incredibly dangerous effects it has on your brain, not just because it can ruin your body forever. It really doesn't work!

Take Away Message

Starving yourself and skipping meals has no long term benefit. On this plan, EAT! It is the only way to change body fat percentage and not just lose weight (healthy tissue). Although it isn't OK to go over your macronutrient needs, it is also just as bad to not eat enough to meet your macronutrient needs. Remember changing body fat percentage isn't losing weight. It is increasing lean tissue and burning fat. You need fuel to do that and food is fuel! EAT what you are supposed to EAT, nothing more, nothing less! Finally, if you fail to complete phase 1 properly by starving yourself, phase 2 and phase 3 WILL NOT WORK!

Six Small Meals a Day

The "Timing" principle of this diet plan is simple, but it's a big one. Let's review the six main reasons why you should be eating six small meals a day:

1. Keeping your insulin response to food steady and low is a major factor in burning fat. We do this by eating foods with a low Glycemic Index and a low Glycemic Load. We also do this by keeping our quantities smaller throughout the day. (six small meals) Dips and spikes in insulin levels also happen when our bodies are either overloaded or deprived of nutrients. Eat steadily with six small meals every day.

2. Starvation is a bad thing. Waiting to eat longer then 3-4 hours starts the body's cannibalistic behavior of destroying lean tissue. This action needs to be avoided by constantly giving your body what it needs to feed healthy tissue in order for it to harvest fat instead. Eat six small meals every day!

3. Feeling starved usually leads to gorging yourself the moment you are face to face with food. It is never good to feel that way. Hunger is different. If you eat every 2-3 hours, you will experience hunger, but never starvation. Eat six small meals every day!

4. You will have a "budget" of macronutrients (fat, carbs, and protein) for the day. You can't eat your entire budget in 1 meal. The excess energy your body doesn't need or use will be stored as fat. By the way, are you going to starve the rest of the day? I personally know some people who eat breakfast and don't eat again until dinner. (Not one of them is lean) Spread your budget of macros throughout the day. So, eat six small meals every day!

5. The process of eating, digestion, absorption and use of food energy takes time. You can't eat a meal at 7:00am and then have a snack at 8:00am. You are still dealing with breakfast. This excess intake will now have to be brought to cells that are already full. You know what that is the blueprint for? Fat storage. Don't snack! Wait 2-3 hours between meals. Eat six small meals every day!

6. Finally, eating small meals helps to shrink your stomach. Over time, you will begin to feel full sooner and have less of a desire or an ability to eat a lot. By the way, people in eating contests do the exact opposite. They train by eating one gigantic

meal a day to expand their stomachs. Now, other than that Japanese guy who eats a million hot dogs and is a complete anomaly, these folks are generally **NOT LEAN!**

If you miss a meal, eat as soon as you can and finish your day accordingly with your next meal 2-3 hours from that time. This can be tricky especially when your next feeding time doesn't coordinate when the rest of the family is eating dinner. It does happen. Don't be discouraged! Do your best. Tomorrow is another day.

Take Away Message

**For all the reasons above and about 20 more...
EAT SIX SMALL MEALS A DAY, 2-3 HOURS APART!**

THE STRATEGIES

The choices we make when it comes to eating are born from thoughts and the understanding we have about food. There are particular concepts and strategies you can employ while on the MacroNutrient Diet that will improve your chances of making better choices.

"Stop giving your mind what it WANTS…and start giving your body what it NEEDS!"

Four Types Of Food

There are really only four types of food to choose from, and only one is the right choice. Here they are:

1. Healthy Food That Promotes Fat Loss

2. Healthy Food The Promotes Fat Gain (biggest mistake)

3. Unhealthy Food That Promotes Fat Loss

4. Unhealthy Food That Promotes Fat Gain

#4. Unhealthy Food That Promotes Fat Gain: Obviously unhealthy food that promotes fat gain is off the list. An example is fast food. Empty calorie food has little to no nutrient density. Refined foods at large quantities are ridiculous. If you find yourself eating this way, you are officially off the wagon.

#3. Unhealthy Food That Promotes Fat Loss: There aren't a lot of these foods, but caffeine, for example, does promote a higher metabolism. Don't fool yourself by skipping a meal and thinking a cup of coffee is the answer. You are probably putting cream and sugar in it anyway which destroys the entire purpose of your little scheme.

Artificial sweeteners like crystal light and Splenda are unhealthy and really are not food. I try to avoid them but on occasion I use Stevia which is a bit more natural. Anyway the idea is to reduce your need for sweets. It's part of the psychology. You will crave them less.

#2. Healthy Food The Promotes Fat Gain: This is the most common mistake people make. Nothing is more disappointing then to hear someone tell me they make a kale, blueberry, strawberry and almond milk shake which is 16 ounces. They say it's healthy and I agree: fresh fruit, non-dairy almond milk, kale. But after finding out they use sweetened almond milk, and have no idea how many berries they put in and are drinking 16 ounces, makes it a fat bomb. It's got a ton of calories and sugar. Remember sugar is sugar is sugar. So the fructose in the fruit and the sugar in the almond milk is the blueprint for fat storage.

The other favorite is the salad with grilled chicken. Healthy, right? Until they put an unknown amount of some sugar filled dressing all over it and it's fat storage time. I will admit it still is a better choice than Burger King, but still not good enough!

I'm not arguing that the foods in this category aren't healthy. I am saying that if you want to change your body composition you need to choose foods from the next category.

#1. Healthy Food That Promotes Fat Loss: Nutrient dense food eaten in certain quantities at certain times. The list of approved items in the fat, protein, and carbohydrates categories are included here on pages 110 - 114.

Take Away Message

The only choice you have in order to get incredible results, is healthy food that burns fat. In the right quantities and eaten at the right times throughout the day, these foods hold the blueprint your body needs to build a leaner you!

How To Cheat

I am going to tell you that if you're going to cheat, you might as well just accept that this eating plan isn't for you. With that said, it does happen. You fall off the wagon and then what? Well most people attempt to create some logic in their head to try and catch up. It's like losing $50,000 at a craps table and thinking it's a good idea to mortgage the house to try to win it back. Cut your losses and move on. Here's what you do:

2-3 hours after your little mishap, start right back on the plan as if it never happened!

Tomorrow is another day. Just don't begin to do it every Saturday night and think you'll be ok. You won't. When you fall just get back up, dust yourself off, forgive yourself, and move on.

Take Away Message

Look, it happens. Don't make a habit of it. Just move on and don't look back!

Eating at Restaurants

Going out to eat can be one of the most difficult and one of the easiest diet related events. However, you need a particular strategy to do this right, and here are a few tips you have to keep in mind.

1. Before going out to dinner remind yourself that it's not the "Last Supper" with Christ and the apostles. It's also not a permission slip to go nuts and "enjoy yourself" because something "tastes good" or you "deserve it."

2. Decide before you go if you will be drinking alcohol. Our advice for this diet is to abstain in general, but one glass of wine with dinner if it adds up to your daily macronutrient equation wouldn't be a crime. Remember, food is associated with alcohol consumption and lowers your guard.

3. The question of the day is always, "What will I select from the menu to eat?" and that can be answered by two separate people with very different motives. You just need to be clear which one of you is ordering. Let me explain.

Whatever you order is going to add up to your daily macros and fit the category of foods we are recommending which will help you burn fat, get leaner and accomplish your goals

or

Whatever you order is going to cause you to exceed your daily macros and include foods we do not recommend which will cause you to store fat, gain weight, and jeopardize your health goals. (p.s. it usually tastes amazing and the mental temptation and experience is usually enough to lead you astray!)

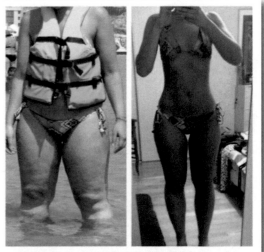

TIP: I sometimes carry a picture of my before and after on my phone. Before I order my meal, I just look at the picture and say which one would I rather be? And what would he order? If you don't have a before and after picture, take a picture of yourself now and then go on the internet and find a picture of the type of body you want. Put them next to one another and keep a digital on your phone. It isn't about vanity but more about the psychology of:

- The unhappy, heavier me ordered what he wanted and it tasted great and he left full, he had no macronutrient responsibility, but ended up like the person on the left.

- The lean me ordered what was good for his body, was even happier when it tasted good, often left the restaurant content but not completely satisfied, had a macronutrient accountability and ended up looking like the person on the right. And here it is again:

"What will I select from the menu to eat?" and that can be answered by two separate people with very different motives. You just need to be clear which one of you is doing the ordering.

So, here is how you do it:

1. Salads are always a great option so long as you remember that you need complete carbs, lean protein and some healthy fat. The dressings, candied walnuts, craisins, orange slices, and tortilla strips are all add-ons that **don't work!** Even within the salad world there are many pitfalls. When in doubt, plain old oil and vinegar on top will do the trick.

2. Avoid pasta all together. Remember whole grain pasta and even things that appear healthy will propel you past your macronutrient requirements with ease. Although you can have pasta on occasion, restaurants aren't the place to roll the dice.

3. Go right to the lean meats like Pork, beef, chicken, fish. Things not smothered in sauce, remember you can have a lean piece of meat smothered in a cream sauce and destroy your plans. Then look at the side it comes with. If it is not a vegetable, complex carbohydrate or a well prepared accompaniment, **swap it out!**

   You can always replace the side with double broccoli, escarole, broccoli rabe, brown rice, mixed vegetables, or any of the approved carbohydrates on the list. Get to know them!

4. If your meal comes with a side of pasta or another refined carbohydrate, swap it with something more appropriate or, tell the waiter or waitress not to even bring it. I know you are paying for it and that someone else at the table may eat it, but that will only tempt you to look at it and think, that's mine. Out of site out of mind.

5. No dessert!!! Do I really need to elaborate here? Coffee, tea, or fruit with low Glycemic Index if they have it and if it fits within your macronutrient equation are O.K. In general, dessert is something to have on a special occasion but know that it is rarely on the approved list of food items.

6. Portion size today is ridiculous. Remember 6 -7 small meals a day. That means at almost every restaurant you will be eating half your meal and saving the rest for later. **Remember Glycemic Load? The higher the indexed food and the higher the Glycemic Load of food (portion size), the greater the insulin and digestive response which equals more fat!**

7. Finally, how a food is prepared will either lead to an unnecessary amount of calories and fat or not. The best and healthiest way food is prepared is as follows:

steamed - grilled - baked - lightly sautéed (still in oil so be careful) - raw - boiled - broiled

8. To drink? Guess: Water with a lemon! Diet sodas should be avoided but they are not the biggest crime against body composition changes. I actually choose a seltzer with a lemon wedge or two.

Take Away Message

The fat you or the lean you will be ordering dinner. Have a game plan going in. Know what your macronutrient needs are. Avoid certain parts of the menu, mix and match your way to a healthy combination, avoid dessert, alcohol and make sure you drink plenty of water (it's free which is a bonus). See the previous section on "How to cheat" if none of this sinks in.

Sabotage or Support

What you think of me is none of MY business!

It is always wonderful when friends, loved ones, and acquaintances are in agreement with and approve of your choices. That however, isn't always the case. If your body has been a certain way for a long period of time, you have to know that not only you, but all the people who know you have come to accept you in that way. (If you wake up one morning and shave all the hair off your head, it will cause a stir amongst everyone who knows you.)

Here is the kicker: after reading this book and adopting this diet, you will have hopefully, changed what you are willing to accept about yourself. Maybe you are tired of being overweight and carrying around excess fat. It's unhealthy. But, this doesn't mean all the other people in your life have accepted that yet.

Believe it or not, losing weight and cleaning up your act is threatening to others. What if you are actually healthier and look better than they do? What does this mean for their own decisions and the work they need to do? What if they are not ready to see you 50 pounds lighter? Believe me, I got a lot of support and even more sabotage. Eventually, people got over it. They did because my body was important to me and I wasn't going to stop this journey. My opinion of my lifestyle outweighed their opinion of my lifestyle.

Now, I am not just talking about your neighbors or co-workers. I am talking about your mom, dad, brothers, sisters, kids, and even your own wife or husband. What if others find you more attractive now and you get attention in a different way? Losing weight and changing your body composition is and will be visible for all to see just like shaving your head bald.

As you change your body composition and begin to lose weight, you will be shocked and amazed that people in your life will either sabotage you or support you. Sadly, the ones closest to you tend to be the sabotagers and the ones further from your inner circle tend to be the supporters. (This isn't always true. Some people are generally just supporters or sabotagers no matter what.) After all, the change in social, physical, and emotional dynamic has a much greater impact on those close to you. You may now want to go out more or dress differently. Change is always a threat to some. They are afraid at some level. Losing weight and getting healthier should only have one response from those close to you and that's love and support.

Either way, it has nothing to do with you. Their opinion is their issue, but they will offer both back handed and rude comments without even batting an eye. So just be prepared. Don't get mad at them or write them off. Explain yourself and your goals and reassure them that what you're doing is good for you and that you would appreciate their support on this difficult journey. Here are a few examples:

Scenario 1:

Husband: "You are getting too thin! I don't like it. Stop doing this, your face looks too thin!"

You: "Uh… OK thanks!"

Scenario 2:

Distant Acquaintance: "Did you lose weight? You look amazing!!!"

You: "Yes, I did. I lost 40 lbs. on the MacroNutrient Diet.(cheap plug) Thank you!

Take Away Message

The point here is that people fear change even if it is good change. Whatever you do, DO NOT ALLOW THIS TO DETER YOU! Don't get angry. In your mind forgive them, for they know not what they do. You are on a mission to succeed and change your life in a positive way. What they think of you is none of your business. Those are their thoughts therefore, it's their business!

The Top Ten Rules To Succeed on The MacroNutrient Diet

The following rules are a list of "must follow" ones on this eating plan. These are non-negotiable and must be adhered to in order for you to maximize the results that are to come. They are each explained individually in the sections to follow.

Rule #1:   Eat Every 2-3 Hours

Rule #2:   Choose Nutrient Dense Food

Rule #3:   Drink Plenty Of Water

Rule #4:   Adhere To Your Math Equation

Rule #5:   No Alcohol (This one can be difficult!)

Rule # 5A: Limit Sugar

Rule #6:   No Snacking, Just Meals

Rule #7:   Your Last Meal Must Be Carbohydrate Free

Rule #8:   Never Skip A Meal

Rule #9:   Accept That Hunger And Cravings Are A Part Of Life

Rule # 10:   Failure Is Not An Option

Rule #1: Eat Every 2-3 Hours (Timing)

Remember the Quality, Quantity, Timing concept? Well, this is all about timing.

TIMING: You must eat no sooner than two hours and no longer than three hours apart (Eat every 2-3 hours only.)

The word snack must be officially eliminated from your vocabulary. **There is no snacking!** Simply 6 meals every 2-3 hours. By meals we are talking about the correct macronutrients in small amounts throughout the day. Recipes and approved macronutrients are listed on pages 110 - 114.

Having emergency meals like prepared protein powders and quest bars in your car or at work are crucial. Not eating begins the blueprint for harvesting lean tissue and slowing fat burning. You must feed muscles to change body fat percentage.

One other important factor here is the idea that we don't want to create a large Glycemic Load. We want to keep our insulin response level throughout the day. When you eat the right foods every 2-3 hours, you keep your cravings down, you prevent yourself from building a huge appetite which causes you to gorge, and you keep your metabolism running non-stop!

Rule #2: Choose Nutrient Dense Food (Quality)

In the previous section nutrient dense vs. empty calorie food, we were able to see that choosing the right food allows you to get the micro and macronutrients your body needs for health and to burn fat. Empty calorie food just sparks the insulin response and starts fat storage.

You will get better over time at choosing these foods at restaurants and in the supermarket. Because of the overwhelming amount of poor food quality everywhere you turn, you must do the due diligence to look at the food label and count your macros as well as looking down the ingredients list to avoid sugar additives. Again, for your benefit we have listed the approved macronutrients on pages 110- 114.

Rule #3: Drink plenty of water

Considering we are mostly made of water and that water is the substance for digestion, cell function and muscle make-up, you need to drink plenty of it.

You need to be drinking water with every meal to aid digestion and absorption of macronutrients and you need to be drinking water between meals. Drinking water helps to curb hunger.

Although non-caloric powders like crystal light are generally not good for you for tons of reasons, if you need to use them for the purposes of fat burning, they are a minor offense.

Just remember, your liver is responsible for over 30% of your resting metabolism. If it is busy filtering poison (alcohol, crystal light, chemicals in diet sodas, etc.), you will be affecting the capacity for you to burn fat!

Rule #4: Adhere To Your Math Equation (Quantity)

If you forget what this means, refer to the chapter on the math on page 46. This is basically what I call Macronutrient accountability. Prior to starting this diet, you were probably unaware of the grams of carbs, fat, and protein you were ingesting. Now, you need to make sure at the end of the day, after you know what your calculated macronutrients are for the day, that you hit those targets. (We will show you how to get these within each phase of the diet in the next chapters) No more and no less than the recommended ranges. No negotiating and no bargaining! Here is an example:

If your macronutrient intakes for the day were:

Fat: **50 - 80g**

Carbs: **140 - 170g**

Protein: **130 - 160g**

Then this is what it might look like to make sure you hit your numbers:

Meal 1	6:30am	- - ½ cup egg whites, 2 Kashi Waffles, ¼ cup fresh Blueberries
Meal 2	9:30am	- Scoop protein powder and 1 cup of unsweetened almond milk as a shake, ½ cup oatmeal with cinnamon
Meal 3	12:30pm	- 2 Scoops protein powder
Meal 4	2:30pm	- 3 oz Grilled Chicken, 1 cup Quinoa, 3 slices avocado
Meal 5	5:30pm	- 3 oz Grilled Salmon, 1 Medium Yam, ½ Cup Roasted Veggies
Meal 6	8:30pm	- 3 oz London Broil, ½ Cup Grilled Veggies

The above example meal plan would provide the following (approximately):

Calories:	1,757	Target: **1,700 - 2,000 Calories**
Fat:	**51g**	Target: **50 - 80g**
Carbs:	**151g**	Target: **140 - 170g**
Protein:	**144g**	Target: **130 - 160g**

Rule #5:   No Alcohol (Quality)

If you are anything like me, then you enjoy alcohol at weddings, parties and with meals. The dietary recommendations for alcohol include 1 beverage per day for women and 2 beverages for men (Normal sizes, not the Chili's 24oz. Sam Adams Seasonal).

But, remember, alcohol has 7 calories per gram which is only 2 calories less than 1 gram of fat (9 calories per gram). It is also an empty calorie as it is not a nutrient dense food but an empty calorie food.

When alcohol is ingested, it must be used by the body as a primary fuel source before the other macronutrients. This doesn't bode well for burning fat. Oh, and one last thing, remember the liver again:

"Your liver will be busy

dealing with the booze

and because of that

no fat will you lose!" ~ me

Rule # 5A: Limit Sugar (Quality)

Sugar is not something that promotes fat loss. If you have not read the cardiovascular surgeon's letter towards the end of the book, make sure you do so. It is clear that sugar can be dangerous over time. A huge amount of products on the market in today's world have added sugar. Check the nutrient labels and be on the lookout for sugar. Over 4-8 grams per serving is usually not for you while on this plan.

On this plan, it is suggested that in your carbohydrate totals for the day, fewer than 15-20 grams are allowed to be sugar.

Rule #6   No Snacking, Just Meals (Quantity & Timing)

This rule relates to the "eating every 2-3 hours" rule. Although some of the quantities of these meals may feel like snacks, they are not. Feeling completely stuffed after a meal isn't something you will experience often. Get used to it, it is normal. Feeling stuffed is really one of your body's warning signs and not a reason to celebrate! Eliminate the word snack from your vocabulary. No seriously, do it now. When someone says would you like a snack, you say, "What the hell is a snack?"

Rule #7   Your Last Meal Must Be Carbohydrate Free (Quality & Timing)

Eating after 8:00pm sounds like a crime in the diet world, but it isn't as long as you eat the right stuff. What would be better than to be feeding muscle while you sleep and keep your metabolism burning as you sleep? Don't skip this meal!

On the other hand, eating empty calories or foods containing any carbs at all is not recommended. For this rule, your last meal at night must contain NO CARBS! Ok, no carbs is tough, but as in the example on page 68, the carbs need to be limited and must come from good sources. Definitely **NO SUGAR!** A carb-free protein shake may be a good idea.

P.S. This is usually when the drinking begins. Now do you see the reason why alcohol and carbs at night are a double whammy? Stay away if getting lean is your mission!

Rule #8   Never Skip a Meal (Timing)

By this time in the book if you still think not eating is a good idea, put this book down and find something else to do. Better to eat than starve when it comes to this type of plan. The rationale that you will be saving calories is also the strategy that prevents you from getting the macronutrients your muscles need to survive. **EAT!!!**

Rule #9:   Accept That Hunger And Cravings Are A Part Of Life

When I begin to eat according to this plan, will I be hungry? Of course! When you don't eat like this don't you also experience moments of hunger? It is a part of being human. The difference is that with macronutrient accountability, you can be rest assured that even if you are hungry, you will be eating again soon and that the math equation for your diet assures you will get what you need, not always what you want.

After all, getting what you want is what got you here. Are you happy? If not, try something different, something that works. There is a bit of suffering, but that too shall pass.

Cravings are negotiable! People crave cigarettes, alcohol, food, sweet things to eat, sex and all sort of other stuff. That is just your mind and subconscious telling you that you'll be happy when you get it. But, that's really a lie. If you get it, guess what happens tomorrow. Your mind is back to convince you again. Fight through them, drink water and move on. This too shall pass. Instead of dessert, sometimes I drink coffee to satisfy the need to be putting something in my mouth. This is tough, but you will be fine!

Rule # 10: Failure Is Not An Option

If you are going to do this, then do it! You owe it to yourself for the next 3-6 months of your life to commit to this whether you like it or not. In the grand scheme of things, it is such a small period of time in your life. Once you begin to see the results I hope you gain the strength to continue on.

Deciding to use this plan is a choice that requires mental toughness! So remind yourself that failure is not an option. Get your macros and move on.

Food is a JOB!

If you want food to be a source of happiness, accept that it is not and find a hobby. Food is a means of survival. It is like a job. It pays the bills so when work is over you can have fun. Like a job, if you love what you do, it's a bonus. If you love the food you are about to eat and it fits the concepts in this book; awesome!

I can tell you that not every meal is satisfying to me. The fact that I would expect it to be is really ridiculous. You mean to tell me every time you eat you are overwhelmed with joy? If you are, I can tell you that you are either overweight or you have enough time and resources to make this happen. It isn't realistic for most people!

You will succeed and change your body composition with the concepts in this book.

FAILURE IS NOT AN OPTION!!!

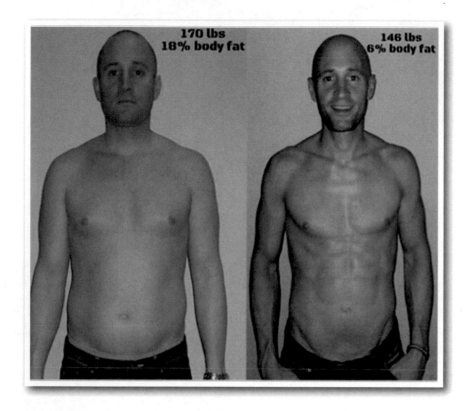

Remember, 4 -5 months, using the concepts in this book, I changed my body in a way I had never done before. You too, will come to know that food is just a blueprint and this book is the guide.

This is not easy and is also not for everyone but, it does work!

WHAT ARE YOU CAPABLE OF?

THE MACRONUTRIENT DIET PLAN:

Three Phases

To summarize, burning fat and getting lean is all about successfully combining the three Principles of: Quality, Quantity, and Timing!   It's six meals a day, eaten 2-3 hours apart, comprised of quality foods, all adding up to the allowed amounts for the day.

1. The diet is made up of three specific phases each building the blueprint and preparing the body for the next phase. Do not alter any stage or you jeopardize the effectiveness of the next phases.

2. The main goal of The MacroNutrient Diet is to know your specific macronutrient grams of carbohydrates, protein , and fat for the day. (i.e. 150g of Carbs, 150g of Protein, and 50g of Fat)

3. You will then create and consume 6 meals a day, each of which contains these macronutrients to reach your limit of carbohydrates, protein, and fat. (Your Macronutrients) You must eat your first meal within the hour you wake up.

4. Do this every day in each specific phase using the concepts discussed in the Quality, Quantity, Timing, and Strategies sections of this book.

Note: Consuming under, or over these macronutrient ranges each day will inhibit your body's ability to burn fat, so we will provide you with a safe range. If you succeed in hitting your macronutrient ranges every day for the duration of this diet you will drastically change your body. It is completely understandable that you will make mistakes, but you must continue to learn and work hard at sticking to the foundations of this diet. Unfortunately, the more rules and strategies you violate, the more you miss your macronutrient ranges, the harder it will be for your body to respond. You will have difficult moments, but it will get easier with time and will eventually become your lifestyle.

Don't count calories, count macronutrients. Know your Macros!

Preparing Each of the Three Phases

1. It's time to start your Three Phase Macronutrient Diet Plan spanning approximately **3-4 months.**

2. Each phase will last approximately **4-6 weeks.**

3. In the beginning of each phase you will need to go to the Macronutrient Calculator at **http://macronutrientcalculator.com** to get your TDEE (caloric intake limit for the day), so you can convert that to your specific, daily macronutrient needs. The process is explained on the following pages.

4. In order to keep the process as simple as possible, and FREE, we are excluding Body fat %. However, a nutrition consultation including body fat measurements is highly recommended and included in all of our in-person consultations.

5. Once you have your macronutrient amounts for grams of carbohydrates, proteins, and fats, you can begin to apply the rules of this diet and plan meals accordingly (sample meals are included on page 115)

6. On pages 140 - 141 there are a blank forms to record the appropriate information for tracking purposes.

7. Take pictures at the beginning, end, and at each phase of the diet. They are inspiring to others and are a great keepsake for your journey! You do tend to forget what you once looked like and because progress is slow, you tend not to see it. Take pictures with the same camera at the same angle in the same lighting in the same outfit. (Better with minimal but appropriate clothing. You will want to show others!)

How to Prepare your Macronutrient Needs for each Phase

Step 1: Go to **//MacronutrientCalculator.com**

NOTE: It is <u>NOT</u> www.macronutrientcalculator.com. There is a link to this calculator on our homepage at www.MacroNutrientDiet.com.

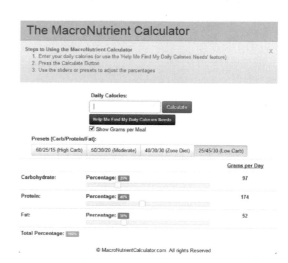

Step 2: Click on the red button that says, "Help me find my daily caloric needs" to get your TDEE (calories)

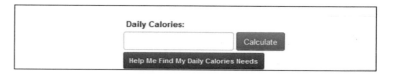

Step 3: Fill out the information on this Daily Caloric Needs Calculator. It is important that you weigh yourself on the same scale and at the same time of the day to keep consistent throughout this process and in each phase.

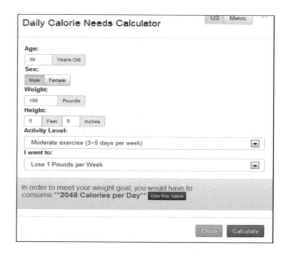

Step 4: Under the Activity level section, click the appropriate level of exercise you plan on performing throughout this program. The less you plan on exercising the lower the caloric needs will be. If you will not be working out at all, click "Little to no exercise." For everyone else, we recommend clicking, "Light exercise (1-3 days per week)" even if you plan on doing a bit more.

Step 5: Under the "I want to:" section, click the amount of pounds to lose per week.

Note: We do not recommend you choose the option, " Lose 2 lbs. per Week."

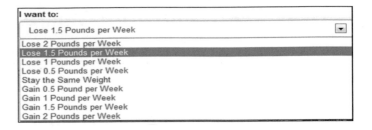

Step 6: After you have completely filled out the information, click the "calculate" button at the bottom right of the page as seen here

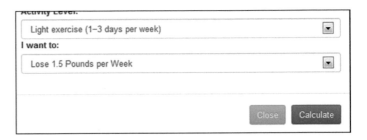

Step 7: If you have completed this form correctly, you should now see a box appear that contains the calories per day. Within that box there is a smaller red box that says," Use this Value." Simply click that button. This will take you back to the Macro calculator, only now, the calories per day will be auto-filled with your caloric needs. It should automatically calculate your macro needs below however, you may need to click the calculate button to the right of the auto-filled calories one more time.

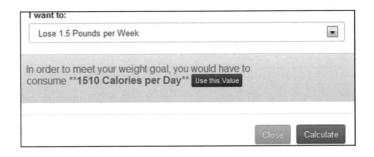

You should now be looking at a screen like the one on the right. At the top of the site is your caloric intake for the day and at the bottom, there is a breakdown of the macronutrients you will need to adhere to as described in the chapters you just read. Congratulations, you have just achieved the first step in your fat loss journey!

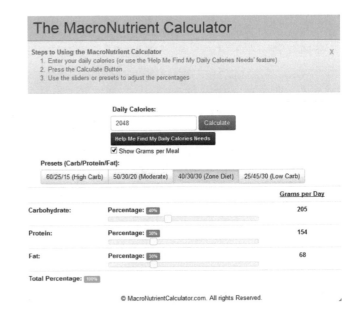

NOTE: The numbers below need to be tailored a bit in order to start phase 1. The macronutrients at this level are not your starting, phase 1 numbers, just your calories are. I will show you how to get your daily macronutrients on the next page.

Take Away Message

The process outlined above is only one of many ways to help you get going. At our one-on-one nutrition consultations, we measure body fat percentage with calipers or tape measurements. We do this because measuring body fat is a far superior way to measure body composition changes. For the purpose of providing you with a FREE way to do this, the above method is the simplest way to go. If you have access to a professional who can calculate your body fat percentage it will be a better way to track changes other than weighing yourself on the scale.

Now it is time to get your macronutrient levels (Your Math Equation)
for Phase 1

Phase 1

In this phase you are going to lose weight, but it is really about changing behavior, and applying all the knowledge you have just gotten throughout this book. It takes time to get accustomed to quality, quantity and timing.

You need to go shopping and be prepared to use and cook with the approved carbohydrates, proteins and fats. These are listed on pages 110 - 114. There is also an Amazon site where you can get supplements, Quest Bars, shaker bottles, complex carbohydrate options, food containers and cooking appliances that are approved, and crucial for succeeding on The MacroNutrient Diet. Because it is an Amazon store, your order over $35 qualifies for free shipping. I would personally wait to start until you have your schedule and foods ready to go! Here is the link: **http://astore.amazon.com/macronutrientdiet-20**

Once you have completed your caloric needs and entered them into the calculator, you will notice a group of presets along the middle of the page as seen here. You will be clicking the 40/30/30 (Zone Diet) option.

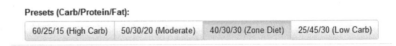

As you can see here in the picture to the right, this would be an example of macronutrient needs for a person who has a daily caloric intake of 1600 calories. Notice at the bottom, it tells you the "Grams per Day" of each of the macronutrients you will need for the first phase of your diet.

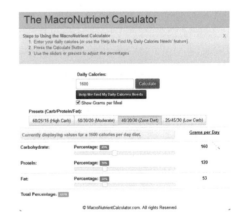

Take Away Message

The process outlined above is only one of many ways to help you get going without a one-on-one consultation.

Your individualized eating plan is based on your measurements and your macronutrients. Depending on your goals, there may be several phases to your plan. **Within each phase (lasting about 4-6 weeks)** your macronutrients will be adjusted to trigger changes in body composition. Fill in your numbers for your Phase 1 Daily Caloric and Macronutrient Totals you achieved in the previous section.

Daily Caloric and Macronutrient Totals

Total daily calories: _____ Range: _____ to _____ calories

(Now put the number you got in the first blank space above. To get your range, subtract 150 from your caloric daily needs and write this in the first "Range" blank space above. Now add 150 to your caloric needs and write this number in the second "Range" blank space above. This is the range you must fall into each day while in phase 1)

Example: 1500 calories per day would be a range of between 1350-1650 calories per day

Total daily Carbs: _____ Range:_____ to _____ grams

Total daily Protein: _____ Range:_____ to _____ grams

Total daily Fat: _____ Range:_____ to _____ grams

(Now put the numbers you got for your macros in the first corresponding macro category above. To get you ranges, subtract 15 from your total daily carbohydrate macro needs and put that number in the first blank "Range" carbohydrate space above. Now add 15 to your total daily carbohydrate macro needs and put that in the second "Range" space above. Do the same for protein and fat)

Example: 160 grams of carbs per day would be a range of between 145-175 grams per day

Total daily macronutrient intake should be evenly spaced out over 6 to 7 meals approx. 2-3 hours apart. It is essential to use lean proteins, complex carbs, and healthy fats to hit your daily macronutrients targets. Use the list of approved Protein, Carbs, and fat on pages 110 - 114 to plan your meals. Use the example meal plan at the end of this phase one plan as a guide for timing of meals and amounts of food per meal.

Remember, calories are made up of the macronutrients: protein, carbohydrates, and fats, each playing crucial roles in the body. The quality, quantity and timing of these macronutrients is key to body composition manipulation! Calories are just a guide. Focus on your macros!

Protein

- Evenly distribute your protein throughout your meals.
- Look for lean sources of protein.
  - O Certain cuts of beef, particularly roasts and ribs are high in saturated fat.
  - O Dark meat chicken tends of have higher saturated fat.
- Consider other macronutrients present in protein sources.
  - O Beans and legumes offer both valuable protein and carbohydrates.
- Keep "emergency" protein handy (at work, when traveling, at the gym, etc.).
  - O Protein bars
  - O Protein shake packets and shaker bottles

Carbohydrates

- READ THE LABELS!–WATCH FOR UNEXPECTED SUGAR!
- The amount of carbohydrates absorbed by your body is considered your "net carbs."
  - O This is easily calculated by subtracting the grams of fiber from the total amount of carbohydrates.
- Seek "whole grain" products. Don't get dooped by labels such as "multi-grain" or "ancient grain."
- Avoid refined carbohydrates.
- With the exception of roots and squash-type vegetables, the carbohydrates in vegetables are negligible—eat rather liberally!
- Spread your carbohydrates out throughout the day, except for your last meal of the day.
- The sugar that you consume during the day (i.e., apple, berries, etc) are best eaten after exercise to help your body quickly replenish glycogen stores in the muscles.

Fats

- Try your best to meet your daily fat through whole, natural sources of fat.
- Use oils sparingly.
- Oils are best consumed at room temperature.
  - O Avoid oils that are solid at room temperature. (ie. butter, margarine)
- Oils differ in heat tolerance. Heat intolerant oils become unhealthy when cooked with, and should be avoided. Look for the following heat tolerant oils:
  - O Avocado, macadamia nut, canola, safflower
- Be careful when eating out. Often, sauces are cooked in butter/oil and contain high amounts of fat and/or sugar.

Water

Water is essential for every function of the body, including fat loss. Water is responsible for nearly 60% of your body weight and makes up about 75% of your muscles. For our purposes, the amount of water to consume is significantly greater than that which is typically recommended

16oz of water with every meal and 16oz between every meal.

Six meals a day is approximately 200oz of water which is about a gallon and half per day (this is tough so do your best)

Avoid carbonated beverages; this will interfere with protein absorption. Avoid juices and most sports drinks, as most are high in high-fructose corn syrup and other sugars. **Avoid Alcoholic beverages**.

Example Meal Layout:

The below example are NOT your numbers. This is just an example!

The following is an example of meals for a day to show you the timing, amounts, and types of food to fulfill your daily total macronutrients in the appropriate manner. This meal plan does not necessarily reflect the exact foods you will be eating or the exact times you will eat them. On page 115 there are several recipes you can choose from. You may also go to our website, www.MacroNutrientDiet.com and click on the links for other recipe ideas. Any foods in a recipe that are not on the approved list should be substituted with the appropriate amount of an approved food.

Meal 1	6:30am	- ½ cup egg whites, 2 Kashi Waffles, ¼ cup fresh Blueberries
Meal 2	9:30am	- Scoop protein powder and 1 cup of unsweetened almond milk as a shake, ½ cup oatmeal with cinnamon
Meal 3	12:30pm	- 2 Scoops protein powder
Meal 4	2:30pm	- 3 oz Grilled Chicken, 1 cup Quinoa, 3 slices avocado
Meal 5	5:30pm	- 3 oz Grilled Salmon, 1 Medium Yam, ½ Cup Roasted Veggies
Meal 6	8:30pm	- 3 oz London Broil, ½ Cup Grilled Veggies

The above example meal plan would provide the following (approximately):

Calories: **1,757**   Target: **1,700 - 2,000 Calories** (You can see you always get your calories when you get the right macros)

Fat: **51g**   Target: **50 - 80g**

Carbs: **151g**   Target: **140 - 170g**

Protein: **144g**   Target: **130 - 160g**

Phase 2

You will start this phase approximately 4-6 weeks after starting phase 1. In this phase your body should be adjusted to timing and eating habits. Your metabolism has changed, you should feel comfortable with what, how much, and how often you are eating. You may need to go back and re-read the book to refresh yourself with the concepts.

By now you should have lost weight and more importantly, if you are working out as prescribed, have changed your body composition. It's time to change the blueprint and your macros to alter the way your body will manipulate and deal with fat. It's also time to alter your workout routine (explained on page 104).

It is time to go back to **http://MacronutrientCalculator.com** and get your macros for phase 2.

Step 3: By this time your weight has changed, so you will need to go back and recalculate your daily caloric needs. It's the red button that says, "Help me find my daily caloric needs." It takes you back to the screen on the right here. Fill out the information on this Daily Caloric Needs Calculator. Again, It is important that you weigh yourself on the same scale and at the same time of the day to keep consistent throughout this process and in each phase.

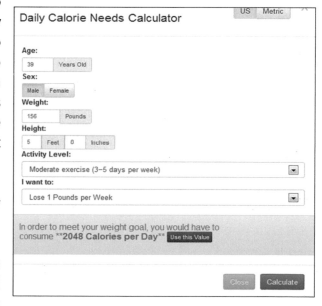

NOTE: The only information that will probably need to be changed is your weight.

Once you completely and correctly fill out the form, hit calculate at the bottom. Then click the red button that says, " Use this Value" This will again take you back to the original screen. (refer to page 75 for the initial detailed explanation of this process.)

Once you have completed your caloric needs and entered them into the calculator, you will notice a group of presets along the middle of the page as seen here. **For Phase 2, you will be clicking the 25/45/30 (Low Carb) option.**

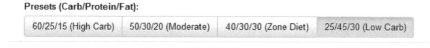

As you can see here, the picture to the right, would be an example of macronutrient needs for a person in Phase 2 who has a daily caloric intake of 1600 calories. Notice at the bottom, it tells you the "Grams per Day" of each of the macronutrients you will need for the second phase of your diet.

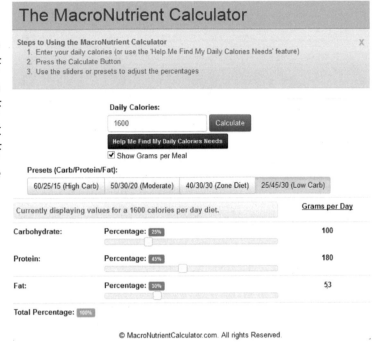

Your individualized eating plan is based on your measurements and your macronutrients. Depending on your goals, there may be several phases to your plan. **Within each phase (lasting about 4-6 weeks)** your macronutrients will be adjusted to trigger changes in body composition. Fill in your numbers for your Phase 2 Daily Caloric and Macronutrient Totals you achieved in the previous section.

Daily Caloric and Macronutrient Totals

Total daily calories: _____   Range: _____ **to** _____ **calories**

(Now put the number you got in the first blank space above. To get your range, subtract 150 from your caloric daily needs and write this in the first "Range" blank space above. Now add 150 to your caloric needs and write this number in the second "Range" blank space above. This is the range you must fall into each day while in Phase 2)

Example: 1500 calories per day would be a range of between 1350-1650 calories per day

Total daily Carbs: _____   Range:_____ **to** _____ **grams**

Total daily Protein: _____   Range:_____ **to** _____ **grams**

Total daily Fat: _____   Range:_____ **to** _____ **grams**

(Now put the numbers you got for your macros in the first corresponding macro category above. To get you ranges, subtract 15 from your total daily Carbohydrate macro needs and put that number in the first blank "Range" carbohydrate space above. Now add 15 to your total daily carbohydrate macro needs and put that in the second "Range" space above. Do the same for protein and fat)

Example: 160 grams of carbs per day would be a range of between 145-175 grams per day

Total daily macronutrient intake should be evenly spaced out over 6 to 7 meals approx. 2-3 hours apart. It is essential to use lean proteins, complex carbs, and healthy fats to hit your daily macronutrients targets. Use the list of approved protein, carbs, and fat on pages 110 - 114 to plan your meals. Use the sample meal plan at the end of this phase one plan as a guide for timing of meals and amounts of food per meal.

Remember, calories are made up of the macronutrients: protein, carbohydrates, and fats, each playing crucial roles in the body. The quality, quantity and timing of these macronutrients is key to body composition manipulation! Calories are just a guide. Focus on your macros!

Protein

- Evenly distribute your protein throughout your meals.
- Look for lean sources of protein.
  - Certain cuts of beef, particularly roasts and ribs are high in saturated fat.
  - Dark meat chicken tends of have higher saturated fat.
- Consider other macronutrients present in protein sources.
  - Beans and legumes offer both valuable protein and carbohydrates.
- Keep "emergency" protein handy (at work, when traveling, at the gym, etc.).
  - Protein bars
  - Protein shake packets and shaker bottles

Carbohydrates

- READ THE LABELS!–WATCH FOR UNEXPECTED SUGAR!
- The amount of carbohydrates absorbed by your body is considered your "net carbs."
  - This is easily calculated by subtracting the grams of fiber from the total amount of carbohydrates.
- Seek "whole grain" products. Don't get dooped by labels such as "multi-grain" or "ancient grain."
- Avoid refined carbohydrates.
- With the exception of roots and squash-type vegetables, the carbohydrates in vegetables are negligible–eat rather liberally!
- Spread your carbohydrates out throughout the day, except for your last meal of the day.
- The sugar that you consume during the day (i.e., apple, berries, etc) are best eaten after exercise to help your body quickly replenish glycogen stores in the muscles.

Fats

- Try your best to meet your daily fat through whole, natural sources of fat.
- Use oils sparingly.
- Oils are best consumed at room temperature.
  - Avoid oils that are solid at room temperature. (ie. butter, margarine)
- Oils differ in heat tolerance. Heat intolerant oils become unhealthy when cooked with, and should be avoided. Look for the following heat tolerant oils:
  - Avocado, macadamia nut, canola, safflower
- Be careful when eating out. Often, sauces are cooked in butter/oil and contain high amounts of fat and/or sugar.

Water

Water is essential for every function of the body, including fat loss. Water is responsible for nearly 60% of your body weight and makes up about 75% of your muscles. For our purposes, the amount of water to consume is significantly greater than that which is typically recommended

16oz of water with every meal and 16oz between every meal.

Six meals a day is approximately 200oz of water which is about a gallon and half per day (this is tough so do your best)

Avoid carbonated beverages; this will interfere with protein absorption. Avoid juices and most sports drinks, as most are high in high-fructose corn syrup and other sugars. **Avoid Alcoholic beverages.**

Example Meal Layout:

The below example are NOT your numbers. This is just an example!

The following is an example of meals for a day to show you the timing, amounts, and types of food to fulfill your daily total macronutrients in the appropriate manner. This meal plan does not necessarily reflect the exact foods you will be eating or the exact times you will eat them. On page 115 there are several recipes you can choose from. You may also go to our website, www.MacroNutrientDiet.com and click on the links for other recipe ideas. Any foods in a recipe that are not on the approved list should be substituted with the appropriate amount of an approved food.

Meal 1	6:30am	- ¾ cup egg whites, 1 Kashi Waffle, ¼ cup fresh Blueberries
Meal 2	9:30am	- Scoop protein powder and 1 cup of unsweetened almond milk as a shake
Meal 3	12:30pm	- 2 Scoops protein powder
Meal 4	2:30pm	- 4 oz Grilled Chicken, ½ cup Quinoa, 3 slices avocado
Meal 5	5:30pm	- 4 oz Grilled Salmon, ½ cup Quinoa, ½ Cup Roasted Veggies
Meal 6	8:30pm	- 4 oz London Broil, ½ Cup Grilled Veggies

The above example meal plan would provide the following (approximately):

Calories:	**1,528**	Target: **1,450 - 1,750 Calories** (You can see you always get your calories when you get the right macros)
Fat:	**54g**	Target: **50 - 80g**
Carbs:	**82g**	Target: **70 - 100g**
Protein:	**165g**	Target: **145 - 175g**

Phase 3

It has now been 8-12 weeks since you started this process and you should notice results by now. You will start phase three 4-6 weeks after starting phase two. In this phase we are going to make the magic happen. We are now going to create a ketogenic blueprint. This is basically getting your body to process fat as your primary fuel source for energy. It Is important to remember that exercise, especially weight training and achieving 60% max heart rate with exercise is happening in this phase.

NOTE: You cannot stay on this phase for more than 8 weeks.

It is time to go back to **http://MacronutrientCalculator.com** and get your macros for phase 3.

Again, as in phase 2, your weight has changed, so you will need to go back and recalculate your daily caloric needs. It's the red button that says, "Help me find my daily caloric needs." It takes you back to the screen on the right here. Fill out the information on this Daily Caloric Needs Calculator. Again, It's important that you weigh yourself on the same scale and at the same time of the day to keep consistent throughout this process and in each phase.

NOTE: The only information that will probably need to be changed is your weight.

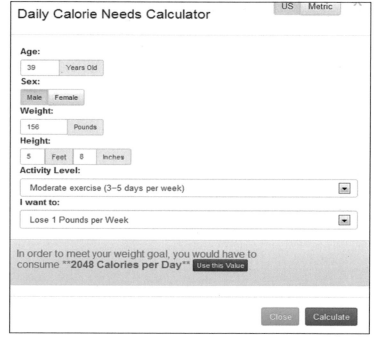

Once you completely and correctly fill out the form, hit calculate at the bottom. Then click the red button that says, " Use this Value" This will again take you back to the original screen. (refer to page 75 for the initial detailed explanation of this process.)

Once you have completed your caloric needs and entered them into the calculator, **you will need to manually change your percentages on the bottom of the macronutrient calculator. Do not use the presets in this phase.**

Slide the carbohydrate bar down to 5%, the protein bar to 50% and the fat bar to 45%.

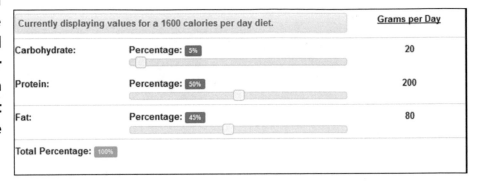

Currently displaying values for a 1600 calories per day diet.		Grams per Day
Carbohydrate:	Percentage: 5%	20
Protein:	Percentage: 50%	200
Fat:	Percentage: 45%	80
Total Percentage: 100%		

As you can see here in this picture, this would be an example of macronutrient needs for a person in Phase 3 who has a daily caloric intake of 1600 calories. Notice at the bottom, it tells you the "Grams per Day" of each of the macronutrients you will need for the third phase of your diet.

Your individualized eating plan is based on your measurements and your macronutrients. Depending on your goals, there may be several phases to your plan. Within each phase (lasting about 4-6 weeks but no longer then 8 weeks!) your macronutrients will be adjusted to trigger changes in body composition. Fill in your numbers for your Phase 3 Daily Caloric and Macronutrient Totals you achieved in the previous section.

Daily Caloric and Macronutrient Totals

Total daily calories: _____ Range: _____ **to** _____ **calories**

(Now put the number you got in the first blank space above. To get your range, subtract 150 from your caloric daily needs and write this in the first "Range" blank space above. Now add 150 to your caloric needs and write this number in the second "Range" blank space above. This is the range you must fall into each day while in Phase 3)

Example: 1500 calories per day would be a range of between 1350-1650 calories per day

Total daily Carbs: _____ Range:_____ **to** _____ **grams**

Total daily Protein: _____ Range:_____ **to** _____ **grams**

Total daily Fat: _____ Range:_____ **to** _____ **grams**

(Now put the numbers you got for your macros in the first corresponding macro category above. To get you ranges, subtract 15 from your total daily Carbohydrate macro needs and put that number in the first blank "Range" carbohydrate space above. Now add 15 to your total daily carbohydrate macro needs and put that in the second "Range" space above. Do the same for protein and fat)

Example: 160 grams of carbs per day would be a range of between 145-175 grams per day

Total daily macronutrient intake should be evenly spaced out over 6 to 7 meals approx. 2-3 hours apart. It is essential to use lean proteins, complex carbs, and healthy fats to hit your daily macronutrients targets. Use the list of approved protein, carbs, and fat on pages 110 - 114 to plan your meals. Use the example meal plan at the end of this phase one plan as a guide for timing of meals and amounts of food per meal.

Remember, calories are made up of the macronutrients: protein, carbohydrates, and fats, each playing crucial roles in the body. The quality, quantity and timing of these macronutrients is key to body composition manipulation! Calories are just a guide. Focus on your macros!

Protein

- Evenly distribute your protein throughout your meals.
- Look for lean sources of protein.
    - Certain cuts of beef, particularly roasts and ribs are high in saturated fat.
    - Dark meat chicken tends of have higher saturated fat.
- Consider other macronutrients present in protein sources.
    - Beans and legumes offer both valuable protein and carbohydrates.
- Keep "emergency" protein handy (at work, when traveling, at the gym, etc.).
    - Protein bars
    - Protein shake packets and shaker bottles

Carbohydrates

- READ THE LABELS!—WATCH FOR UNEXPECTED SUGAR!
- The amount of carbohydrates absorbed by your body is considered your "net carbs."
    - This is easily calculated by subtracting the grams of fiber from the total amount of carbohydrates.
- Seek "whole grain" products. Don't get dooped by labels such as "multi-grain" or "ancient grain."
- Avoid refined carbohydrates.
- With the exception of roots and squash-type vegetables, the carbohydrates in vegetables are negligible—eat rather liberally!
- Spread your carbohydrates out throughout the day, except for your last meal of the day.
- The sugar that you consume during the day (i.e., apple, berries, etc) are best eaten after exercise to help your body quickly replenish glycogen stores in the muscles.

Fats

- Try your best to meet your daily fat through whole, natural sources of fat.
- Use oils sparingly.
- Oils are best consumed at room temperature.
    - Avoid oils that are solid at room temperature. (ie. butter, margarine)
- Oils differ in heat tolerance. Heat intolerant oils become unhealthy when cooked with, and should be avoided. Look for the following heat tolerant oils:
    - Avocado, macadamia nut, canola, safflower
- Be careful when eating out. Often, sauces are cooked in butter/oil and contain high amounts of fat and/or sugar.

Water

Water is essential for every function of the body, including fat loss. Water is responsible for nearly 60% of your body weight and makes up about 75% of your muscles. For our purposes, the amount of water to consume is significantly greater than that which is typically recommended

16oz of water with every meal and 16oz between every meal.

Six meals a day is approximately 200oz of water which is about a gallon and half per day (this is tough so do your best)

Avoid carbonated beverages; this will interfere with protein absorption. Avoid juices and most sports drinks, as most are high in high-fructose corn syrup and other sugars. **Avoid Alcoholic beverages.**

Example Meal Layout:

The below example are NOT your numbers. This is just an example!

The following is an example of meals for a day to show you the timing, amounts, and types of food to fulfill your daily total macronutrients in the appropriate manner. This meal plan does not necessarily reflect the exact foods you will be eating or the exact times you will eat them. On page 115 there are several recipes you can choose from. You may also go to our website, www.MacroNutrientDiet.com and click on the links for other recipe ideas. Any foods in a recipe that are not on the approved list should be substituted with the appropriate amount of an approved food.

Meal 1	6:30am	- 1 cup egg whites, 1 whole egg
Meal 2	9:30am	- 1 Scoop protein powder and 1 cup of unsweetened almond milk as a shake
Meal 3	12:30pm	- 2 Scoops protein powder
Meal 4	2:30pm	- 5 oz Grilled Chicken, 3 slices avocado
Meal 5	5:30pm	- 5 oz Grilled Salmon, ½ Cup Roasted Veggies
Meal 6	8:30pm	- 5 oz London Broil, ½ Cup Grilled Veggies

The above example meal plan would provide the following (approximately):

Calories:	**1,492**	Target: **1,250 - 1,550 Calories** (You can see you always get your calories when you get the right macros)
Fat:	**70g**	Target: **50 - 80g**
Carbs:	**18g**	Target: **0 - 30g**
Protein:	**180g**	Target: **160 - 190g**

Maintenance Phase

You have just completed all three phases of The MacroNutrient Diet, now what? Your body and health should have undergone a tremendous transformation if you adhered to the principles of this plan. But this is really a lifestyle. You can put yourself back on and off it when you choose. You have all the tools at your disposal. Below is what we suggest for maintaining your nutrition plan.

At the completion of phase 3, simply go back to the macronutrient calculator online and get your TDEE or total daily caloric limit for the day as described in the previous chapters. This time you will need to select the activity level and adjust that if you plan on changing your workouts. You also need to select the **"Stay the Same Weight"** option under the **"I want to:"** section and calculate.

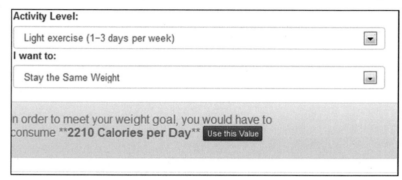

Once you click, "Use this value" , we suggest you put yourself back on phase 1 which is the 40/30/30 (Zone Diet). You may also use the 50%/30%/20% (Moderate) however, you are free to choose as you wish. You may also put yourself back on the diet as often as you want. Just figure out if you want to lose weight, stay the same, or gain weight. Then use the calculator to get your daily macronutrient needs. It's that simple!

Presets (Carb/Protein/Fat):

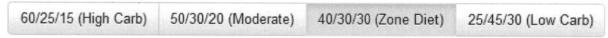

| 60/25/15 (High Carb) | 50/30/20 (Moderate) | 40/30/30 (Zone Diet) | 25/45/30 (Low Carb) |

If you got this far, you should now have a firm grasp on how to manipulate your weight and body composition. You have all the tools to be your own diet expert. Know your macros!

Congratulations and Good Luck!

P.S. Please send us your pictures and your story at info@MacroNutrientDiet.com. You may just be the inspiration for someone else to change his/her life.

THE MACRONUTRIENT DIET PLAN:

The Exercise

There are literally thousands of exercise programs on the market. Because exercise is really only about 20% of the process of getting lean, it's not worth getting injured on some elaborate exercise regimen. This section includes the process by which you should introduce exercise into your plan. It starts simple, with a focus on technique and posture. This is a diet book, so if you feel you have an exercise program that accomplishes the goals we recommend, then you are more than welcome to do it your way. **However, for the diet portion of this book.... DON'T ALTER IT!**

Your Exercise Plan for Phase 1

Similar to the diet which has several phases, your exercise plan also has several phases. In phase 1 you will need to learn and practice correct exercise technique. That includes understanding posture, as well as proper application of this posture into an exercise setting. The reality is that exercise is one of the leading causes of injury in home and gym workouts. You will need to learn how to avoid this problem and how to start exercising the RIGHT way. In general, the first 2-4 weeks of any exercise program is really just neuromuscular education. So, learning the right way to exercise is crucial in order to avoid derailing your program with an injury. Remember the 70:20:10 rule from page eight? Although integral in your long term success, exercise is only 20% of the solution anyway.

Before we begin to look at the phases of exercise you must first understand that **hours of cardio are NOT the way to burn fat!** Fat burning and building muscle comes from specific forms of exercise.

High Intensity Interval Training (THIS IS IT!) Basically, the combination of high intensity exercise followed by resting periods has been shown to significantly burn more fat than "cardio." This is a scientific fact. Feel free to do all the research you want, but I'll save you the time. It is also why you see the emergence of p90x, Crossfitt, and T25 at gyms.

This idea excuses you from hours on the treadmill. But you will need to gain muscle mass which is metabolically active long after your work out is over. Secondly, you will be improving your body fat percentage, resulting in more muscle, less fat. Finally, if done correctly, you can create a cardiovascular experience without running.

"But I'll Get Bulky!"

This is the first thing women say when I discuss resistance training but it simply isn't true! Since women don't produce any real significant testosterone, any muscle you build will only really create definition and turn your metabolically active muscle tissue into fat burning machines, even at rest! Cardio doesn't really do that!

Take Away Message:

You don't need to spend hours walking, running, or anything of the sort! The most effective exercise should take you less than an hour 2-4 days a week and must include interval training and resistance training. It will get you into the fat burning zone and keep you there long after you're done exercising. It's science, trust it! I also highly recommend a heart rate monitor. I have several listed on the Amazon site. In my opinion, the simpler the better!

Remember that the initiation of an exercise plan starts with education of both your mind and body. This is the preparation phase. As a physical therapist I have seen far too many people sidelined from the wrong exercise all in an attempt to lose weight. For this reason, I created:

www.StopExercising.com

Simply go to www.StopExercising.com, and download the FREE, 1 hour instructional DVD. This will start to lay the foundation for exercising correctly and more importantly help prevent an injury which will most likely also derail your diet.

In the video, you will learn how to set your posture with exercise using Total Body Posture™, implement the Three Step Exercise Technique ™, learn and master the top upper and lower gym resistance machines, understand the correct form of doing an abdominal crunch, and finally, learn the most effective top 10 stretches for your entire body.

The video isn't sexy, it's educational. It also isn't mandatory, but highly recommended. It only gets more complicated from here, so starting with poor exercise knowledge and technique will catch up with you! I see it every day!

Step 3: If joining a gym isn't your thing, I have a FREE in-home exercise program for you. Simply go to www.StopExercising.com, click the "Blog" section at the top. Once there, at the bottom of the first blog post, it says:

==> CLICK HERE to download your FREE Workout

You simply click that statement and print the .pdf file. There are also links on purchasing the resistance band and other items needed for the program. (I recommend starting with a medium band, but 1 of each of the light, medium and hard bands will allow for adjusting your workout as you progress.)

Step 4: On the next page, I have attached the workout. It is an alternating day program between upper and lower body. Remember this is phase 1. It's about neuromuscular education, learning movement, posture and waking up your muscles and orthopedic system to the stress of exercise. It is NOT about building Rome in a day.

Step 5: You will start this routine when you start your diet, although you can certainly start earlier. This phase is designed to prepare your body for phase 2. Complete this routine 2-4 days a week for about 4 weeks alternating between upper and lower body.

Remember the 70:20:10 rule from page eight? Well, you need the 10% rest days so fit them in every 1-2 work-out days. Please contact us if you need help in completing this phase, however, all the information you need is available at StopExercising.com and on the DVD. Good Luck!

Stop Exercising Until You See This!

www.StopExercising.com

PHASE 1 EXERCISE PROGRAM

If you currently have a workout plan, just apply Total Body Posture™ and the Three Step Exercise Technique™, taught in this DVD, to all of your exercises. Always remember your body's warning signs and

NEVER EXERCISE IF YOU HAVE PAIN!

If you have never worked out before or just need to get back to the basics, the following workout is a simple way to ensure that you are getting a balanced diet of exercise. Completing each section of this workout the RIGHT way, is thoroughly explained in the DVD. Even if you have been exercising for years, there is a lot to learn, so you may need to go back and review the DVD to ensure your success.

For this exercise program, complete all of the exercises in the "Lower Body" workout. Then, on another day, at your next workout, complete all of the exercises in the "Upper Body" workout. Now, the next time you exercise, you will simply alternate back to the "Lower Body" workout. Continue this alternating pattern every workout. This routine ensures that you get cardiovascular training and resistance training, as well as the recommended stretching at each workout. You will also allow your muscles to recover on off days. This alternating schedule ensures you satisfy the national recommendations for exercise.

Stop Exercising Until You See This!

www.StopExercising.com

PHASE 1 EXERCISE PROGRAM
DAY 1

LOWER BODY

Lower Body Warm Up

(Approximately 5 minutes)

Bike · Treadmill · Elliptical, etc.

Lower Body Stretch

(Hold the stretch for 30 seconds and repeat on each side)

Calf · Hamstring · Quadriceps · Piriformis · Groin

Lower Body Resistance Training

(30 to 40 repetitions until fatigue)

Leg Extension · Leg Curl · Leg Press · Calf Press · Hip Abduction · Hip Adduction

---

Cardiovascular Training

(Approximately 30 minutes at your target heart rate)

Bike · Treadmill · Elliptical, etc.

Heart Rate between 60% and 80% of your calculated maximum heart rate. The chart to find your personal target heart rate is in the cardiovascular section of the DVD.

Abdominal Training

Abdominal training can be done on either workout day. Just like any other muscle in your body, you should allow 24-48 hours of rest between abdominal workouts. Complete repetitions of the abdominal crunch shown in the DVD until you reach fatigue. Rest for 30 seconds to a minute and repeat for 3-4 more sets.

Stop Exercising Until You See This!

www.StopExercising.com

PHASE 1 EXERCISE PROGRAM

DAY 2

UPPER BODY

Upper Body Warm Up
(Approximately 5 minutes)

Upper Body Cycle

Upper Body Stretch
(Hold the stretch for 30 seconds and repeat on each side)

Upper Trap · Rotator Cuff · Posterior Capsule · Wrist Flexor & Extensor · Pectoral

Upper Body Resistance Training
(30 to 40 repetitions until fatigue)

Seated Row · Overhead Shoulder Press · Biceps Curl · Triceps Extension · Lat Pull Down

Chest Press · Pec Deck · Reverse Pec Deck

Cardiovascular Training
(Approximately 30 minutes at your target heart rate)

Bike · Treadmill · Elliptical, etc.

Heart Rate between 60% and 80% of your maximum heart rate. The chart to find your personal target heart rate is in the cardiovascular section of the DVD.

Abdominal Training

Abdominal training can be done on either workout day. Just like any other muscle in your body, you should allow 24-48 hours of rest between abdominal workouts. Complete repetitions of the abdominal crunch shown in the DVD until you reach fatigue. Rest for 30 seconds to a minute and repeat for 3-4 more sets.

Phase 1 Flow Sheet

Here is a blank flow sheet for you to use to track your workouts. Date the top and fill in the amount of weight and number of reps for each exercise completed.

UPPER BODY	LOWER BODY

NAME _____

	AGE	HR		AGE	HR
	30 – 39 :	115 – 140		60 – 69 :	95 – 120
	40 – 49 :	105 – 135		70 – 79 :	90 – 110
	50 – 59 :	100 – 125			

Step 2: Set yourself

Keep your feet forward and in line with your knees.
Keep your hips straight. Keep your pelvis in neutral.
Keep your shoulders **DOWN & BACK!**

Exercise Date

Warm-Up & Cardio

Arm Bike Fwd: Bkwd:
Treadmill
Eliptical
Bike

Stretches/Other

Circuit Machines

Step 1: Set the machine

S = Seat   L = Leg   C = Chest   B = Back

1) Leg Ext   S: L:
2) Leg Curl   S: L:
3) Multi Hip   L:
4) Hip ADduction: *Sit First*
5) Hip ABduction: *Open First*
6) Leg Press   S:
7) Seated Row   S: C:
8) Shoulder Press S:
9) Biceps Curl   S: C:
10) Triceps Ext   S: B:
11) Rear Delt / Pec Deck S:
12) Chest Press   S:
13) Lat Pulldown (Standing)

Your Exercise Plan for Phase 2 & 3

Now that phase one of your exercise program is complete, you should have an understanding of the basics for posture control, weight training, crunches and stretching. Most importantly doing them RIGHT! As we ramp up here a bit, these techniques serve to reduce your risk of injury. Remember, listen to your body's warning signs. After all, we are trying to change our bodies, not damage them.

One of the original programs that began the interval training idea was Bill Phillip's "Body For Life" routine. I have modified it a bit but the principles are the same. I have copied the instructions from the Body For Life site so you understand the routine. Visit **www.BodyforLife.com** for more detailed information on this recommendation.

Remember, in this plan you get cardio, resistance training, abdominal work, variation, rest and all within 50-60 minutes for the upper body and only 50-60 minutes for the lower body. Most importantly, this helps build lean muscle, keeps you in your fat burning zone and keeps it streamlined. The same rules apply for alternating scheduling. You will do the upper body workout one day and then at the next workout you complete the lower body routine. Cardio, if you desire, is done on the days in between the upper and lower body days.

Take Away Message:

The concepts here are basically the same however we are now ramping it up a bit. Use variety of exercises within each body part. Whatever you do, never sacrifice form or posture with exercise. Follow the principles from www.StopExercising.com and the DVD to significantly reduce your risk for injury.

Official Body-*for*-LIFE Weight-Training Plan

www.BodyforLife.com

(Upper & Lower Body)

- Weight train intensely, three times per week on alternating days with aerobic exercise three times per week. Make sure to hit your "high points" during your workout.

- Alternate training the major muscles of the upper and lower body.

- Perform two exercises for each major muscle group of the upper body.

- Select one exercise and conduct five sets with it, starting with a set of 12 reps, then increasing the weight and doing 10 reps, adding more weight and doing 8 reps, adding more weight for 6 reps. Then reduce the weight and do 12 reps. Immediately perform another set of 12 reps for that muscle group using the second selected exercise.

- For each muscle group, rest for one minute between the first four sets. Then complete the final two sets with no rest in between, wait two minutes before moving on to your next muscle group, complete this pattern five times for the upper body training experience and four times for the lower body training experience.

- Always plan your training before hand.

- Record all your weightlifting exercises in a journal indicating the exercise selected and weight lifted.

www.BodyforLife.com

Official Body-for-LIFE Cardio-Training Plan

Cardio workouts are indispensable to an effective training program and general good health. By definition, cardio workouts can be any exercise—jogging, running, biking, swimming, elliptical machine, climbing stairs, even jumping rope—that raises and maintains your heart rate over a predetermined amount of time. By doing so, you strengthen your heart and lungs and lower your resting heart rate, which means that over time the same effort that produced a 10-minute mile will produce a 9-minute mile. Cardio workouts burn fat. And cardio fitness is what gives you endurance and the ability to persist in sports and in life.

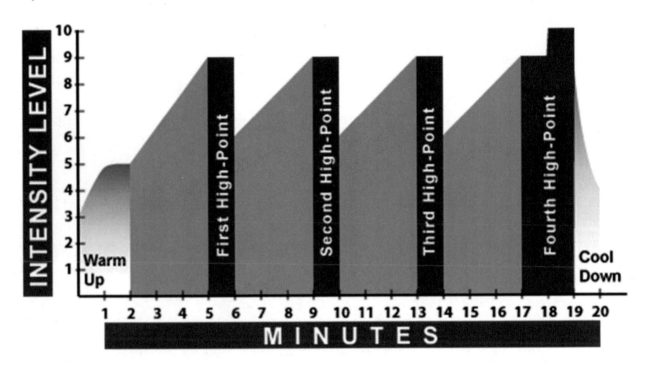

20-Minute Aerobics Solution™ – The Official Body-for-LIFE Cardio Plan

1. Warm up the first 2 minutes at Intensity Level 5

2. Minutes 2-3 move from Intensity Level 5 to 6

3. Minutes 4-5, 6-10 and 11-14 work your way from Intensity Level 6 to Level 9, maintain for one minute.

4. Minutes 15-19 work your way from Intensity Level 6 to Level 10 (High Point at Level 10), maintain for one minute.

5. Minute 20 cool down to Intensity Level 5 for one minute.

Remember, I achieved the results I got without cardio. My cardio was from the intensity of the upper and lower body strength training routines. However, cardio is good for you and generally should be included.

Go to www.BodyforLife.com for more detailed information on this exercise plan and blank flow sheets for tracking your workouts

Take Away Message

The world of exercise is beyond the original scope of this book however necessary to achieve optimal results. Exercise is dangerous and an injury is sure to derail your progress.

You are more than welcome to choose your own plan however, I highly recommend that you adhere to the principles found at www.StopExercising.com.

THE MACRONUTRIENT DIET PLAN:

The Resources

Serving Size

It's not always easy to know exactly what a serving size really looks like and not everyone can carry measuring spoons with them while eating or preparing food. Below is a quick guide you can use to determine the portion size of something while eating or cooking.

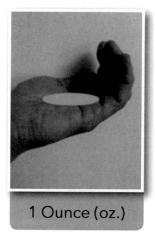

1 Ounce (oz.)

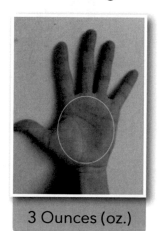

3 Ounces (oz.)

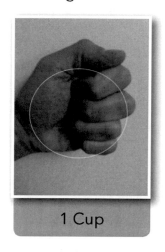

1 Cup

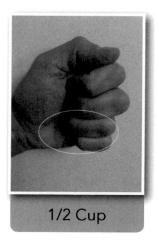

1/2 Cup

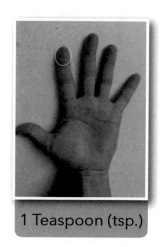

1 Teaspoon (tsp.)

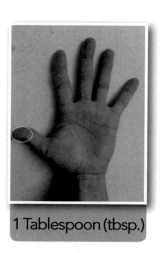

1 Tablespoon (tbsp.)

List of Acceptable Macronutrients

Complex Carbohydrates

Lean Proteins

Healthy Fats

This list can also be used as a grocery list. The majority of the meals you make will involve these foods due to the many factors discussed in this book. And remember, the majority of these foods will be found in the periphery of the supermarket. Only venture down the middle aisles for specific foods. No browsing!

Please Note: Some foods, specifically fruits and vegetables, if eaten whole, will be counterproductive to changing body composition. For instance, the amount of sugar in a whole apple is often too much. Therefore, if you choose to eat an apple, you will need to eat part of an apple. As in label reading, you must check serving size and adjust the amount eaten to meet your macronutrient needs for the day. For this reason, we have included the key below:

Key (for carbohydrates)

"Safer" for fat burning needs.

Proceed with caution. Keep portion size small.

List of Acceptable Complex Carbohydrates

	Serving Size	Cal	Fat	Protein	Carbs	Sugar	Fiber	GI	GL
Grains									
Quinoa	1/2 cup cooked	115	2	4	21	0	2	53	13
Brown Rice	1/2 cup cooked	107	<1	3	22	0	2	50	16
Wheat Berries	1/2 cup cooked	150	<1	6	32	0	6	40	11
Freekeh	1/2 cup cooked	130	1	8	26	1	4	43	13
Farro	1/2 cup cooked	170	1	7	35	0	5	40	12
Cous Cous	1/2 cup cooked	88	0	3	18	0	1	65	9
Oatmeal	1/2 cup cooked	73	1	3	13	0	2	60	13
Steel Cut Oats	1/2 cup cooked	150	3	5	27	1	4	40	11
Ezekiel Bread	1 slice	80	<1	4	15	0	3	35	6
Ezekiel English Muffin	1/2 muffin	80	<1	4	15	0	3	35	6
100% Whole Wheat Wrap	1 wrap	80	3	7	14	0	6	40	6
Kashi 7 grain waffle	2 waffles	150	5	4	24	3	7	65	
Beans/legumes									
Black Beans	1/2 cup cooked	109	<1	7	20	0	8	35	6
Red Kidney Beans	1/2 cup cooked	109	<1	6	20	0	8	35	6
Cannellini	1/2 cup cooked	109	<1	7	20	0	8	30	6
Garbonzo	1/2 cup cooked	110	2	7	20	0	8	35	6
Lentils	1/2 cup cooked	115	0	9	20	0	8	30	6
Fruits									
Blackberries	1/4 cup	15	0	0	3.5	2	2	25	2
Blueberries	1/4 cup	20	0	0	5.5	3.75	1	25	3
Raspberries	1/4 cup	16.25	0	0	3.75	1	2	25	1
Strawberries	1/2 cup	25	0	0	6	3.5	1.5	25	2
Cherries, sweet	1/2 cup	49	0	0	12	10	1.5	25	4
Avocado	half	163	15	2	9	<1	7	10	2
Apple	1 large apple	130	0	0	34	25	5	35	6
Grapefruit	1/2 grapefruit	60	0	0	15	11	2	25	<3
Orange	1 medium	80	0	0	19	14	3	35	4
Pear	1 medium	100	0	0	26	16	6	30	4

List of Acceptable Complex Carbohydrates

	Serving Size	Cal	Fat	Protein	Carbs	Sugar	Fiber	GI	GL
Vegetables									
Arugala	1/2 cup	10	0	1	1	0	0	15	0
Asparagus	5 spears	25	0	2	4	2	2	15	0
Bell Pepper	1 medium	30	0	1	7	4	2	15	2
Broccoli	1 medium stalk	45	0	5	8	3	5	15	2
Brussel Sprouts	4 sprouts	40	0	2	6	2	3	15	3
Escarole	1 1/2 cup	15	0	1	3	0	2	15	0
Green Beans	3/4 cup	25	0	1	5	2	3	15	2
Kale	1 1/2 cup	50	0.5	3	1	0	2	15	0
Leaf Lettuce	1 1/2 cup	15	0	1	4	2	2	15	0
Onion	1 medium	60	0	2	14	9	3	15	4
Spinach	1 1/2 cup	40	0	2	10	0	5	15	0
Summer Squash/Zucchini	1 medium	30	0	2	7	4	2	15	2
Butternut Squash	2/3 cup	40	0	1	11	2	2	51	3
Corn	1 medium ear	80	0	3	18	5	3	55	10
Sweet Potato	1 medium	130	0	2	33	7	4	50	11
Tomato	1 medium	35	0	1	7	4	1	50	2

List of Acceptable Proteins

(Meats should be 97% lean or better for maximal results)

	Serving Size	Cal	Fat	Protein	Carbs	Sugar	Fiber	GL
Beef								
London Broil	3 oz	150	4.5	25	0	0	0	0
Porterhouse	3 oz	170	7	24	0	0	0	0
Sirloin	3 oz	160	7	24	0	0	0	0
T-Bone	3 oz	170	7	24	0	0	0	0
Tenderloin/Filet	3 oz	170	8	24	0	0	0	0
Chicken								
Chicken Breast	3 oz	120	<1	28	0	0	0	0
Drumstick	3 oz	160	9	20	0	0	0	0
Thigh (no skin)	3 oz	140	7	19	0	0	0	0
Chicken breast, canned	1 can, 5 oz.	230	10	32	0	0	0	0
Turkey								
Breast/Tenderloin	3 oz	110	1	25	0	0	0	0
Fish								
Salmon	3 oz	175	10	19	0	0	0	0
Tilapia	3 oz	108	3	21	0	0	0	0
Tuna, canned	1 can	220	5	41	0	0	0	0
Tuna, filet	3 oz	156	5	25	0	0	0	0

List of Acceptable Fats

	Serving Size	Cal	Fat	Protein	Carbs	Sugar	Fiber	GL
Nuts								
Almonds	1/4 cup	207	18	8	7	1	4	2
Cashews	1/4 cup	150	12	5	8	2	1	2
Peanuts	1/4 cup	215	19	9	6	1	3	2
Pecans	1/4 cup	171	18	2	3.5	1	2	2
Walnuts	1/4 cup	164	16	4	3	<1	1.5	2
Seeds								
Pumpkin	1/4 cup	160	14	7	5	0	1	2
Sunflower	1/ cup	170	15	7	6	1	3	2
Other								
Oil (all varieties)	1 tbsp	120	14	0	0	0	0	0
Eggs	1 large egg	74	5	6	0	0	0	0
Almond Milk (Unsweetened)	1 cup	30	2.5	1	2	0	1	0
Avocado	half	163	15	2	9	<1	7	2

NOTE: Cinnamon, hot sauces, pickles, vinegar, mustard, spices, and herbs are all calorie free and can absolutely be used to enhance flavor. Just check the nutrient label before using to make sure.

Sample Recipes

Putting it all Together

Recipes

Putting It All Together

Now that you understand the concept behind using macronutrients to manipulate your body composition, you are presented with the challenge of actually putting it into practice. Whereas this may seem like a daunting task, it really is simple. By adhering to a few basic principles, you will be able to prepare simple and flavorful meals that meet your macronutrient needs. This in turn, will empower you to succeed in making permanent dietary lifestyle changes, rather than fail with a transient diet.

Principles for easy meal preparation:

1. The fundamental elements for any meal consist of: lean protein and complex carbohydrates.

2. Essential fats are often incorporated in sources of lean protein, specifically fish.

   a. Natural sources of fats such as nuts, seeds, avocados, and oils (sparingly) can serve as additions to recipes when daily fat intake is low.

3. Other ingredients including appropriate fruit, vegetables, herbs/seasoning should be considered nutrient-dense, flavor-enhancers.

   a. Fruit should be used in extreme moderation, simply due to their potential impact on blood sugar.

   b. Appropriate vegetables, herbs and seasoning can be used more liberally.

4. Supplementation is a great tool for eating meals on the go but should not be used for more than half of your six meals a day.

Strategies for Success:

1. Plan your meals in advance.

2. Cook for multiple days.

3. Precook large quantity of grains for the week.

4.   Use frozen produce. Otherwise, pre-cut/wash your produce for the week.

5.   Always practice good food hygiene when handling meats of any kind.

On the following page there are some sample meals and recipes to put it all together. Understand that all meals can be altered in order to meet your macronutrient needs and taste. Furthermore, the types of lean protein and complex carbohydrates can be substituted. Just keep in mind, the specific profile for each food source is different, because that will ultimately affect the quantity of each ingredient.

On the very last page of this book, there is a blank macronutrient worksheet that you can photocopy and use to plan recipes and meals so you maintain your macronutrient accountability. You can also visit our Amazon store to find some of the approved products for this diet.

http://astore.amazon.com/macronutrientdiet-20

We have also created a new recipe book including over 100 approved MacroNutrient Diet recipes for you to choose from. There are plenty of options for breakfast, lunch, and dinner. We have also gone ahead and completed the macronutrient worksheet for each recipe so you can accurately track the macronutrient content of each meal. This "must have" recipe book can be found on our website at

www.MacroNutrientDiet.com

Breakfast

Pepper and Onion Omelet

Food item	Serving Size	Calories	Fat	Protein	Carbs	Sugar	Fiber
Peppers, diced	1 tbsp	< 5	0	0	0	0	0
Onions, diced	1 tbsp	< 5	0	0	0	0	0
Egg white	½ cup	63	0	13	0	0	0
Cooking spray	¼ sec	0	0	0	0	0	0
Total		68	0	13	0	0	0

Egg White and Tomato Sandwich

Food item	Serving Size	Calories	Fat	Protein	Carbs	Sugar	Fiber
Egg white	½ cup	63	0	13	0	0	0
Cooking spray	¼ sec	0	0	0	0	0	0
Tomato	1 slice	4	0	0	1	.5	0
Toasted Ezekiel English Muffin	1 muffin	160	1	8	30	0	6
Total		227	1	21	31	.5	6

Protein Packed Peanut Butter Oatmeal with Almonds

Food item	Serving Size	Calories	Fat	Protein	Carbs	Sugar	Fiber
Rolled oats	½ cup	73	1	3	13	0	2
PB2 Peanut Powder	2 tbsp	45	1.5	5	5	1	2
Almonds, diced	2 tbsp	82	8	2	1	0	1
Protein Powder (Nitro fusion)	1 scoop	120	2	21	4	4	0
Total		320	12.5	31	23	5	5

Apple-Walnut Cinnamon Oatmeal

Food item	Serving Size	Calories	Fat	Protein	Carbs	Sugar	Fiber
Rolled oats	½ cup	73	1	3	13	0	2
Apple, diced	¼ apple	32	0	0	8	6	1
Walnuts, diced	2 tbsp	82	8	2	1	0	1
Cinnamon, ground	Sprinkle	0	0	0	0	0	0
Total		187	9	5	21	6	3

Blueberry Pecan Oatmeal

Food item	Serving Size	Calories	Fat	Protein	Carbs	Sugar	Fiber
Rolled oats	½ cup	73	1	3	13	0	2
Blueberries	¼ cup	15	0	0	3.5	2	2
Pecans, diced	2 tbsp	85.5	9	1	2	0	1
Total		173.5	10	4	18.5	2	5

Strawberry-Mint Steel Cut Oats

Food item	Serving Size	Calories	Fat	Protein	Carbs	Sugar	Fiber
Steel Cut Oats	½ cup	150	3	5	27	1	4
Strawberry	½ cup	25	0	0	6	1.5	3.5
Fresh mint	pinch	0	0	0	0	0	0
Total		175	3	5	33	2.5	7.5

"Black and Blue" Kashi 7 Grain Waffles (waffles with black and blueberry syrup)

Food item	Serving Size	Calories	Fat	Protein	Carbs	Sugar	Fiber
Kashi 7 Grain Waffle	2 waffle	150	5	4	24	3	7
"Black and blue" syrup	½ cup	35	0	0	9	6	3
Total		185	5	4	33	6	10

**Syrup is made by slowly reducing fresh berries and water over low heat.

Lunch

Chicken Wrap with Roasted Peppers and Arugula

Food item	Serving Size	Calories	Fat	Protein	Carbs	Sugar	Fiber
Chicken breast, sliced	3 oz	120	.5	28	0	0	0
Arugula	½ cup	3	0	0	2	0	0
Roasted Red Peppers, sliced	¼ cup	22	0	0	2	<1	<1
Whole wheat wrap	1 wrap	80	3	7	14	0	6
Total		225	3.5	35	16	<1	7

Turkey Burger on Ezekiel English Muffin with Reduced Sugar Ketchup

Food item	Serving Size	Calories	Fat	Protein	Carbs	Sugar	Fiber
Ground Turkey Breast	3 oz	110	1	25	0	0	0
Leaf lettuce	½ cup	5	0	0	1	0	1
Reduced Sugar Ketchup	1 tbsp	5	0	0	1	1	0
Ezekiel Bread English Muffin	1 muffin	160	1	8	30	0	6
Total		280	2	33	32	1	7

Spinach Salad with Grilled Chicken, Cannellini Beans, and Dijon Mustard Vinaigrette

Food item	Serving Size	Calories	Fat	Protein	Carbs	Sugar	Fiber
Chicken breast, sliced	3 oz	120	.5	28	0	0	0
Spinach	3 cups	80	0	2	10	0	5
Cannellini Beans	½ cup	109	0	7	29	0	8
Dijon Mustard Vin.	To taste	30	0	0	0	0	0
Total		339	.5	37	39	0	13

London Broil with Freekah and Steamed Broccoli							
Food item	Serving Size	Calories	Fat	Protein	Carbs	Sugar	Fiber
London Broil, sliced	3 oz	160	7	24	0	0	0
Broccoli	1 cup	45	.5	5	8	3	5
Freekeh	½ cup	130	1	8	26	1	4
Total		335	8.5	37	34	4	9

Jon's Tuna Fish Sandwich with Apple, Celery, and Walnuts							
Food item	Serving Size	Calories	Fat	Protein	Carbs	Sugar	Fiber
Tuna, canned	1 can	60	0	13	0	0	0
Apple, diced	¼ apple	32	0	0	8	6	1
Celery, diced	½ stalk	5	0	0	1	0	.5
Walnuts, chopped	¼ cup	164	16	4	3	<1	1.5
Leaf lettuce	½ cup	5	0	0	1	0	1
Canola Mayo	1 tbsp	5	0	0	1	1	0
Ezekiel Bread	1 slice	80	1	4	15	0	6
Salt, Pepper, Onion Flakes	To taste	0	0	0	0	0	0
Total		351	17	21	29	8	10

Dinner

Chicken or Steak Fajitas Platter with Quinoa and Black Beans							
Food item	Serving Size	Calories	Fat	Protein	Carbs	Sugar	Fiber
Chicken breast, sliced	3 oz	120	.5	28	0	0	0
Peppers, sliced	½ pepper	15	0	1	7	4	2
Onion, sliced	¼ onion	15	0	0	3	3	1
Quinoa and Black Beans	1/4 cup each	129	1	7	25	1	5
Avocado	½ whole	25	2.5	0	1	0	1
Hot Sauce	To taste	0	0	0	0	0	0
Total		304	4	36	36	8	9

Turkey Tenderloin with Rosemary-Butternut Squash Farro and Roasted Asparagus							
Food item	Serving Size	Calories	Fat	Protein	Carbs	Sugar	Fiber
Turkey tenderloin	3 oz	110	1	25	0	0	0
Butternut squash, diced	2/3 cup	40	0	1	11	2	2
Farro	½ cup	85	0	3	17	0	3
Rosemary	Dash	0	0	0	0	0	0
Asparagus	5 spears	25	0	2	4	2	2
Total		260	1	31	32	4	7

Chicken with Roasted Spinach-Artichoke-Tomato Blend over Brown Rice							
Food item	Serving Size	Calories	Fat	Protein	Carbs	Sugar	Fiber
Chicken breast, sliced	3 oz	120	.5	28	0	0	0
Spinach	3 cups	80	0	2	10	0	5
Artichoke hearts	¼ cup	50	0	2	4	1	2
Tomato, diced	½ whole	16	0	0	3.5	2	1
Brown Rice	½ cup	1.7	1	3	22	0	2
Total		373	1.5	35	39.5	3	10

Supplements

(Shakes & Quest Bars)

While there is no substitute for whole foods, supplementation affords us the opportunity to have a quick and convenient meal. With all the various supplements on the market, it is rather easy to create a meal that meets your macronutrient needs. At the same time, it is just as easy to create a counterproductive meal with supplements. In order to make supplements taste good, manufacturers produce them with disproportionate macronutrients and large quantities of sugar. Therefore, prior to taking a supplement, read the nutrition facts.

The following concepts are important to review prior to creating a meal via supplements.

1. *Carb vs. Carb Restriction.* Recently, more and more protein supplements have been developed with the carbohydrate-restricted dieter in mind. However, there are times where you will want to add complex carbohydrates to your shake. Waxymaize, is one such carbohydrate supplement that can be added to meet your carbohydrate needs and can be found on our Amazon store.

2. *Water vs. Almond Milk.* In general, water is the best thing to make your shake from. At times, almond milk is an acceptable substitute that makes shakes thicker and creamier. When you choose almond milk to make a shake, ensure that is it sugar-free and does not have unnecessary additives such as carrageenan or xanthan gum. ShopRite's Unsweetened Vanilla Almond Milk is our personal choice.

3. *Animal vs. Plant Protein.* Protein is found in a variety of animal and plant sources. Therefore, there are a variety of protein supplements. The most common ones use whey, casein, soy and a blend of plant-based proteins. Depending on your goals, time of consumption, body sensitivities, etc,.–you might chose one over the other. Again, these options and recommendations are on our Amazon store.

Here's an example of 3 different protein shake recipes and a Quest Bar example:

Vanilla Raspberry with Waxymaize							
Food item	Serving Size	Calories	Fat	Protein	Carbs	Sugar	Fiber
Plant Fusion Protein Powder	1 scoop	120	2	21	4	4	0
Almond milk	2 cups	60	5	0	0	0	0
Raspberries	1/4 cup	16	0	0	3.5	1	2
Waxymaize	1 scoop	140	0	0	40	0	0
Ice	6 cubes	0	0	0	0	0	0
Total		336	7	21	47.5	5	2

Peanut Butter Chocolate							
Food item	Serving Size	Calories	Fat	Protein	Carbs	Sugar	Fiber
Plant Fusion Protein Powder (Chocolate)	1 scoop	120	2	21	4	4	0
Almond milk	2 cups	60	5	0	0	0	0
PB 2 Powdered Peanut Butter	2 tbsp	45	1.5	5	5	1	2
Total		225	8.5	26	9	5	2

French Vanilla Coffee							
Food item	Serving Size	Calories	Fat	Protein	Carbs	Sugar	Fiber
Plant Fusion Protein Powder (Vanilla)	1 scoop	120	2	21	4	4	0
Iced Coffee (plain)	2 cups	0	0	0	0	0	0
Total		120	2	21	4	4	0

Quest Bar							
Food item	Serving Size	Calories	Fat	Protein	Carbs	Sugar	Fiber
Quest Bar (Peanut Butter)	1 bar (60g)	210	1.5	20	21	2	17
Total	60 g	210	1.5	20	21 (Only 4g net carbs)	2	17

Products To Buy

There are lots of products that claim to be healthy but remember we are looking for foods that are healthy and cause our bodies to burn fat. I have put together an Amazon.com store and included things that are approved for this eating plan. Simply go to the web site link provided. Remember it's through Amazon and I have attempted to included all items that qualify for FREE shipping after you spend $35 or more. On the top left of the site, the very first category is "GETTING STARTED". You will at least need these products to start the MacroNutrient Diet.

HERE IS THE LINK:

http://astore.amazon.com/macronutrientdiet-20

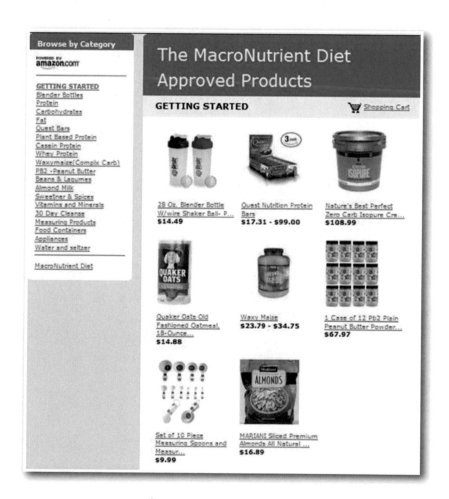

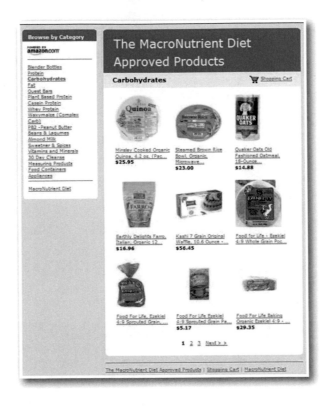

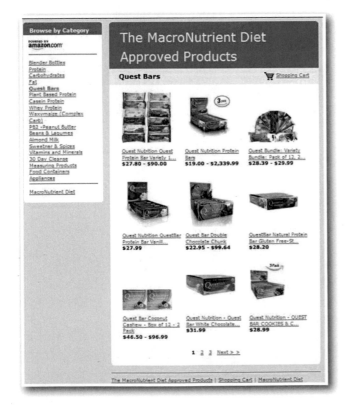

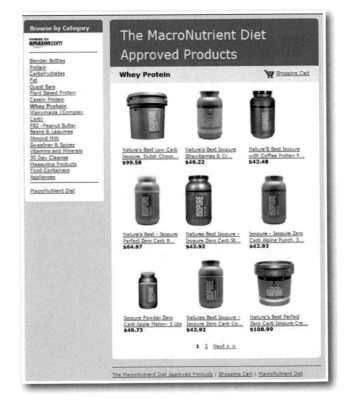

WHAT REALLY CAUSES HEART DISEASE

(Inflammation caused by sugar and omega-6)

by Dr. Dwight Lundell - from: PreventDisease

We physicians with all our experience, "know how" and authority often acquire a rather large selfishness that tends to make it hard to accept we are wrong. So, here it is. I openly admit to being mistaken. As a heart surgeon with 25 years experience, having done more than 5,000 open-heart surgeries, today is my day to right the wrong with medical and scientific proof.

I trained for many years with other prominent physicians labeled "opinion makers." Bombarded with scientific literature, continually attending education seminars, we opinion makers insisted heart disease resulted from the simple fact of elevated blood cholesterol.

The only accepted therapy was prescribing medications to lower cholesterol and a diet that severely restricted fat intake. The latter of course we insisted would lower cholesterol and heart disease. Deviations from these recommendations were considered heresay and could quite possibly result in malpractice.

It Is Not Working!

These recommendations are no longer scientifically or morally defensible. The discovery a few years ago that inflammation in the artery wall is the real cause of heart disease is slowly leading to a paradigm shift in how heart disease and other chronic ailments will be treated.

The long-established dietary recommendations have created epidemics of obesity and diabetes, the consequences of which dwarf any historical plague in terms of mortality, human suffering and dire economic consequences.

Despite the fact that 25% of the population takes expensive statin medications and despite the fact we have reduced the fat content of our diets, more Americans will die this year of heart disease than ever before.

Statistics from the American Heart Association show that 75 million Americans currently suffer from heart disease, 20 million have diabetes and 57 million have pre-diabetes. These disorders are affecting younger and younger people in greater numbers every year.

Simply stated, without inflammation being present in the body, there is no way that cholesterol would accumulate in the wall of the blood vessel and cause heart disease and strokes. Without inflammation, cholesterol would move freely throughout the body as nature intended. It is inflammation that causes cholesterol to become trapped.

Inflammation is not complicated – it is quite simply your body's natural defense to a foreign invader such as a bacteria, toxin or virus. The cycle of inflammation is perfect in how it protects your body from these bacterial and viral invaders. However, if we chronically expose the body to injury by toxins or foods, a condition occurs called chronic inflammation. Chronic inflammation is just as harmful as acute inflammation is beneficial.

What thoughtful person would willfully expose himself repeatedly to foods or other substances that are known to cause injury to the body? Well, smokers perhaps, but at least they made that choice willfully.

The rest of us have simply followed the recommended mainstream diet that is low in fat and high in polyunsaturated fats and carbohydrates, not knowing we were causing repeated injury to our blood vessels. This repeated injury creates chronic inflammation leading to heart disease, stroke, diabetes and obesity.

Let me repeat that: The injury and inflammation in our blood vessels is caused by the low fat diet recommended for years by mainstream medicine.

What are the biggest culprits of chronic inflammation? Quite simply, they are the overload of simple, highly processed carbohydrates (sugar, flour and all the products made from them) and the excess consumption of omega-6 vegetable oils like soybean, corn and sunflower that are found in many processed foods.

Take a moment to visualize rubbing a stiff brush repeatedly over soft skin until it becomes quite red and nearly bleeding. You kept this up several times a day, every day for five years. If you could tolerate this painful brushing, you would have a bleeding, swollen infected area that became worse with each repeated injury. This is a good way to visualize the inflammatory process that could be going on in your body right now.

Regardless of where the inflammatory process occurs, externally or internally, it is the same. I have peered inside thousands upon thousands of arteries. A diseased artery looks as if someone took a brush and scrubbed repeatedly against its wall. Several times a day, every day, the foods we eat create small injuries compounding into more injuries, causing the body to respond continuously and appropriately with inflammation.

While we savor the tantalizing taste of a sweet roll, our bodies respond alarmingly as if a foreign invader arrived declaring war. Foods loaded with sugars and simple carbohydrates, or processed with omega-6 oils for long shelf life have been the mainstay of the American diet for six decades. These foods have been slowly poisoning everyone.

How does eating a simple sweet roll create a cascade of inflammation to make you sick?

Imagine spilling syrup on your keyboard and you have a visual of what occurs inside the cell. When we consume simple carbohydrates such as sugar, blood sugar rises rapidly. In response, your pancreas secretes insulin whose primary purpose is to drive sugar into each cell where it is stored for energy. If the cell is full and does not need glucose, it is rejected to avoid extra sugar gumming up the works.

When your full cells reject the extra glucose, blood sugar rises producing more insulin and the glucose converts to stored fat.

What does all this have to do with inflammation? Blood sugar is controlled in a very narrow range. Extra sugar molecules attach to a variety of proteins that in turn injure the blood vessel wall. This repeated injury to the blood vessel wall sets off inflammation. When you spike your blood sugar level several times a day, every day, it is exactly like taking sandpaper to the inside of your delicate blood vessels.

While you may not be able to see it, rest assured it is there. I saw it in over 5,000 surgical patients spanning 25 years who all shared one common denominator – inflammation in their arteries.

Let's get back to the sweet roll. That innocent looking goody not only contains sugars, it is baked in one of many omega-6 oils such as soybean. Chips and fries are soaked in soybean oil; processed foods are manufactured with omega-6 oils for longer shelf life. While omega-6s are essential -they are part of every cell membrane controlling what goes in and out of the cell – they must be in the correct balance with omega-3s.

If the balance shifts by consuming excessive omega-6, the cell membrane produces chemicals called cytokines that directly cause inflammation.

Today's mainstream American diet has produced an extreme imbalance of these two fats. The ratio of imbalance ranges from 15:1 to as high as 30:1 in favor of omega-6. That's a tremendous amount of cytokines causing inflammation. In today's food environment, a 3:1 ratio would be optimal and healthy.

To make matters worse, the excess weight you are carrying from eating these foods creates overloaded fat cells that pour out large quantities of pro-inflammatory chemicals that add to the injury caused by having high blood sugar. The process that began with a sweet roll turns into a vicious cycle over time that creates heart disease, high blood pressure, diabetes and finally, Alzheimer's disease, as the inflammatory process continues unabated.

There is no escaping the fact that the more we consume prepared and processed foods, the more we trip the inflammation switch little by little each day. The human body cannot process, nor was it designed to consume, foods packed with sugars and soaked in omega-6 oils.

There is but one answer to quieting inflammation, and that is returning to foods closer to their natural state. To build muscle, eat more protein. Choose carbohydrates that are very complex such as colorful fruits and vegetables. Cut down on or eliminate inflammation- causing omega-6 fats like corn and soybean oil and the processed foods that are made from them.

One tablespoon of corn oil contains 7,280 mg of omega-6; soybean contains 6,940 mg. Instead, use olive oil or butter from grass-fed beef.

Animal fats contain less than 20% omega-6 and are much less likely to cause inflammation than the supposedly healthy oils labeled polyunsaturated. Forget the "science" that has been drummed into your head for decades. The science that saturated fat alone causes heart disease is non-existent. The science that saturated fat raises blood cholesterol is also very weak. Since we now know that cholesterol is not the cause of heart disease, the concern about saturated fat is even more absurd today.

The cholesterol theory led to the no-fat, low-fat recommendations that in turn created the very foods now causing an epidemic of inflammation. Mainstream medicine made a terrible mistake *when it advised people to avoid saturated fat in favor of foods high in omega-6 fats. We now have an epidemic of arterial inflammation leading to heart disease and other silent killers.*

What you can do is choose whole foods your grandmother served and not those your mom turned to as grocery store aisles filled with manufactured foods. By eliminating inflammatory foods and adding essential nutrients from fresh unprocessed food, you will reverse years of damage in your arteries and throughout your body from consuming the typical American diet.
~ Dr. Dwight Lundell

Get Started Today or Contact Us

Thank you for taking the time to read this book. I sincerely hope you have taken away information that will further your journey to a leaner and healthier body. But, now it's time to give you the opportunity to do something about it.

Steven Covey, the author of the bestselling book, The 7 Habits of Highly Effective People, once wrote,

"Knowledge is NOT power... applied Knowledge is power!"

You just read all the information necessary to change your body composition, it's time to apply!

Now that we have just given you this great information for FREE, don't' simply give your copy to someone else. If you know anyone interested in a FREE nutrition education and a diet that works to burn fat, send them to our website at:

www.MacroNutrientDiet.com

We can be reached at:

info@MacroNutrientDiet.com

The MacroNutrient Diet

Recipes:

www.MacroNutrientDiet.com

(The MacroNutrient Diet approved recipe book)

Approved Products:

astore.amazon.com/
macronutrientdiet-20

Macronutrient Calculators:

http://macronutrientcalculator.com
www.iifym.com

Glycemic Index:

www.montignac.com

Nutrient information and labels:

www.nutritiondata.self.com
www.caloriecount.com
http://ndb.nal.usda.gov/

iPHONE APP: FOODUCATE

Exercise:

www.StopExercising.com
www.BodyforLife.com

Scientific Research:

www.hsph.harvard.edu/nutritionsource/
www.ajcn.nutrition.org

Body Fat calculator App:

FatCaliper+

(Use the U.S. Navy Non-Caliper Method)

Apps:

FOODUCATE
(highly recommended for scanning products and for nutrient data)
Fitness Calculator
(Use the U.S. Navy, Non-Caliper Method)
MacroCalc
Calorie Count
FatCaliper+
(Use the US Navy Non-Caliper Method)
My Fitness Pal
(Make sure you manually set your macronutrient percentages to match the phase of the diet you are in.)

Before and After Photos

Phase 1

Phase 2

Phase 3

Body Composition Analysis

Date: _____

Phase 1 ☐   **Phase 2** ☐   **Phase 3** ☐

Name: _____   Age: _____   Height: _____ ' _____ " Weight: _____

Email: _____ Cell # _____   BMI: _____   Exercise Frequency: _____

Female Girth	Female Caliper	Male Girth	Male Caliper
Neck: _____ in	Triceps: _____ mm	Neck: _____ in	Chest: _____ mm
Abdomen: _____ in	Thigh: _____ mm	Waist _____ in	Abdomen: _____ mm
Hip: _____ in	Suprailiac: _____ mm		Thigh: _____ mm

Fat Mass: _____ lbs

Lean Mass: _____ lbs

% Body Fat: _____ %

MALE

Age	Excellent	Very good	Good	Fair	Poor
19-24	<11	11.1 - 15	15.1-23	19.1-23	>23
25-29	<13	13.1 - 17	17.1-20	20.1-24	>24
30-34	<15	15.1 - 18	18.1-22	22.1-25	>25
35-39	<16	16.1 - 19	19.1-23	23.1-26	>26
40-44	<18	18.1 - 21	21.1-24	24.1-27	>27
45-49	<19	19.1 - 22	22.1-25	25.1-28	>28
50-54	<20	22.1 - 23	23.1-26	26.1-29	>29
55+	<20	20.1 - 24	27.1-30	27.1-30	>30

FEMALE

Age	Excellent	Very good	Good	Fair	Poor
19-24	<19	19.1-22	22.1-25	25.1-30	>30
25-29	<19	19.1-22	22.1-25	25.1-30	>30
30-34	<20	20.1-23	23.1-26	26.1-31	>31
35-39	<21	21.1-24	24.1-28	28.1-32	>32
40-44	<23	23.1-26	26.1-29	29.1-33	>33
45-49	<24	24.1-27	27.1-31	31.1-34	>34
50-54	<27	27.1-31	31.1-34	34.1-37	>37
55+	<28	28.1-31	31.1-34	34.1-38	>38

- **Weight:** Try to do this right after waking up in the morning

- **Waist:** Measure at naval

- **Hips:** (females only): measure at the fullest point

- **Neck:** Measure just above the adams apple

Research

Gross, A.M., et. Al. (2013) Effects of diet macronutrient composition on body composition and fat distribution during weight maintenance and weight loss. *Obesity. 21(6):* 1139-42.

Kaiser, K.A., et. Al. (2014) Increased fruit and vegetable intake has no discernible effect on weight loss: a systematic review a meta-analysis. *Am J Clin Nutri.*

La Bounty, P.M., et. Al. (2011) International Society of Sports Nutrition position stand: meal frequency. *J Int Soc Sports Nutr 8(4).*

Magkos, F., Avraniti, F., Zampelas, A. (2003) Organic food: nutrition food or food for thought? A review of the evidence. *Int J Food Sci Nutr.* 54(5): 357-71.

Palupi, E., Janavegara, A., Ploeger, A., Kahl, J. (2012) Comparison of nutritional quality between conventional and organic dairy products: a meta-analysis. *J Sci Food Agric. 92(14):* 2774-81.

Speliman, F.A., Azadbakht, L. (2014) Weight loss maintenance: A review on dietary strategies. *J Res Med Sci. 19(3):* 268-75.

Thomas ,D.E., Elliott, E.J., Baur, L. (2007) Low Glycaemic Index or low Glycaemic Load diets for overweight and obesity. *Cochrane Database Syst Rev (3).*

Take Away Message

These are just a few relevant research articles to support the strategies with this eating plan. We encourage you to continue your own independent research and lifelong learning about diet and the food you eat.

Meal Macronutrient Worksheet

Calculate your daily macronutrients per meal per day

Name: _____

Date: _____ / _____ / _____

Meal 1							Time:_____
Food item	**Serving**	**Calories**	**Fat**	**Protein**	**Carbs**	**Sugar**	**Fiber**
Meal 1 Total							

Meal 2							Time:_____
Food item	**Serving**	**Calories**	**Fat**	**Protein**	**Carbs**	**Sugar**	**Fiber**
Meal 2 Total							

Meal 3							Time:_____
Food item	**Serving**	**Calories**	**Fat**	**Protein**	**Carbs**	**Sugar**	**Fiber**
Meal 3 Total							

The MacroNutrient Diet

Meal 4   Time:_____

Food item	Serving	Calories	Fat	Protein	Carbs	Sugar	Fiber
Meal 4 Total							

Meal 5   Time:_____

Food item	Serving	Calories	Fat	Protein	Carbs	Sugar	Fiber
Meal 5 Total							

Meal 6   Time:_____

Food item	Serving	Calories	Fat	Protein	Carbs	Sugar	Fiber
Meal 6 Total							

DAILY TOTALS	Calories:	Fat:	Protein:	Carbs:	Sugar:	Fiber:

Made in the USA
San Bernardino, CA
14 September 2016

38880653R00081